*Toward Mindfulness and Recovery of your
Diet, Lifestyle, Health, and Youthfulness*

BIOLOGICAL

YOUTH

THE FIRST BOOK IN THE
TOTAL RECOVERY SERIES

TODD EWING, PHD

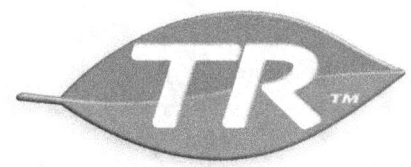

Conceived, written, and illustrated by Todd Ewing, PhD

ISBN-13: 978-1535584456
ISBN-10: 1535584459
Printed in the United States of America

ACKNOWLEDGMENTS

My children Alex, Isaac, Elijah, and Sophie,
for their curiosity, love, and support.

My wife Tara,
for the inspiration to live healthy in my adult years.
For editing, proofreading, and checking all my blindspots.
And most of all, for love and support.

My father and my brother,
for successfully managing type 1 diabetes
and for the inspiration to live healthy in my early years.

CONTENTS

BIOLOGICAL YOUTH

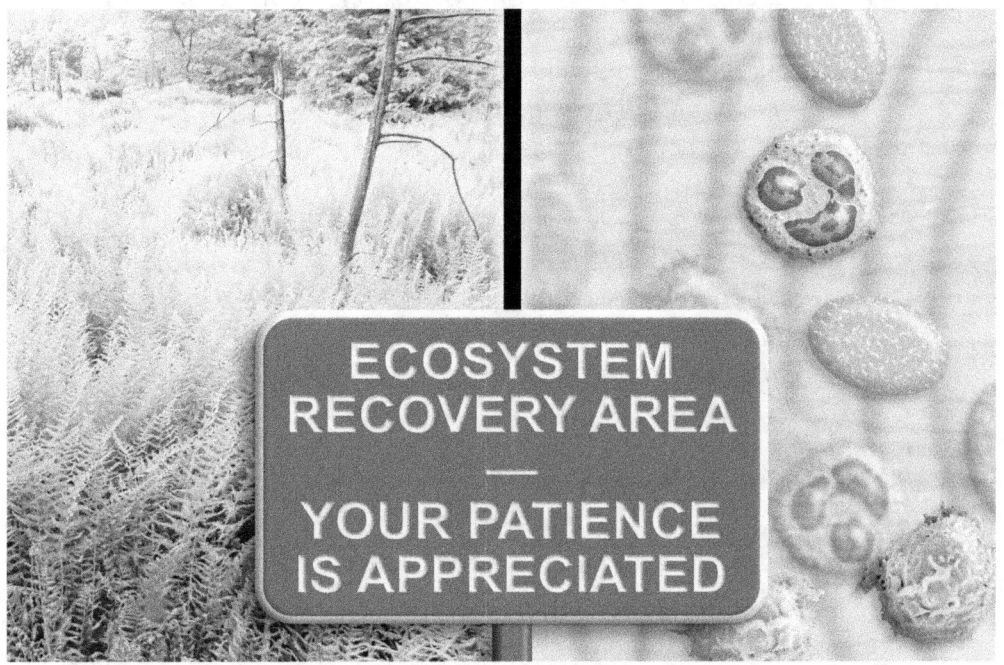

ECOSYSTEM
RECOVERY AREA
—
YOUR PATIENCE
IS APPRECIATED

Ecosystem recovery nurtures rejuvenation and youthfulness.

Total Recovery — or TR — offers us a new way to think about our health that enhances our mindfulness. TR helps us visualize the cells in our bodies as living entities in a cell ecosystem — much like animals and plants in a natural ecosystem. TR helps us visualize how each of our daily activities affects our cell ecosystem. And, each day, as we develop our mindfulness, we can improve the healthiness of our lifestyle, and we can help our cell ecosystem enter a state of recovery.

Total Recovery provides a Theory of Biological Youth which is derived from the total fitness of the body. Total fitness represents the **resilience** of our cell ecosystem to every typical physiological stress. As our total fitness increases, our cell ecosystem enters a state of repair and rejuvenation. With sustained rejuvenation, we can recover our biological youth.

For completeness, the Theory relates biological age to the total frailty of the body. Frailty is the opposite of fitness. Total frailty represents the **vulnerability** of our cell ecosystem to every typical physiological stress. As our total frailty increases, our cell ecosystem enters a state of erosion. With prolonged erosion, we increase our biological age, and we lose our biological youth.

In this chapter, we examine the following topics:
- *Total fitness and the five fitnesses.*
- *The Duke study of biological age.*
- *The Dimmer Switches of Fitness.*
- *The UCLA study of reversing Alzheimer's.*
- *The Theory of Biological Youth.*
- *The traditional theory of aging.*
- *Fitness and frailty.*
- *The total fitness exam.*
- *Review.*
- *Imagine*

TOTAL FITNESS AND THE FIVE FITNESSES

Total fitness represents everything that must go right in our bodies. It is composed of five different fitnesses — metabolic, circadian, microbial, immune, and mental fitness. We're all aware of physical fitness — what TR calls metabolic fitness. Many of us, however, overlook the other four fitnesses.

Even the word "fitnesses" as a plural sounds strange to us. We're used to hearing about "fitness," but not "fitnesses." Total Recovery is attempting something bold by getting us to consider both "total fitness" as a singular and "the five fitnesses" as a plural. It's like how we consider "total color" as a singular and "the many colors" as a plural.

We can imagine total fitness as a beam of pure white light and Total Recovery as an optical prism that splits total fitness into the five fitnesses. The five fitnesses have always been part of total fitness. We've just never thought about them separately.

Each of the five fitnesses represents the resilience of our cell ecosystem to particular stresses on the body. Each fitness is strengthened by different parts of the recovery lifestyle which we examine in *Chapter Seven: Recovery Lifestyle*. Partial loss of any one fitness leads to particular disorders and diseases. Complete loss of any one fitness will eventually lead to death by natural causes.

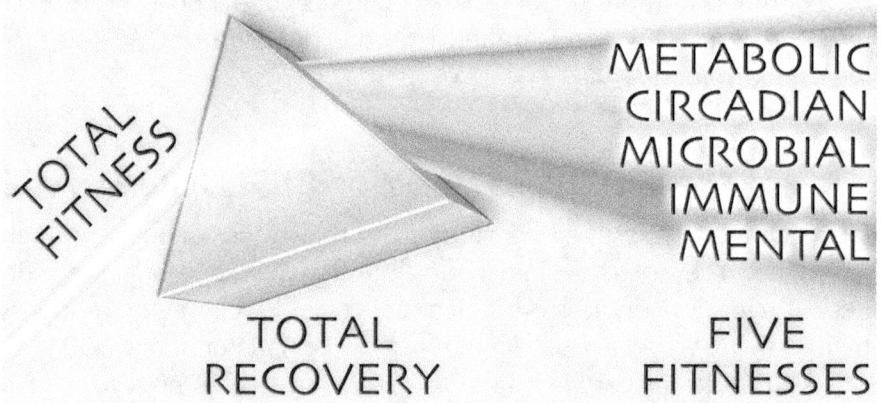

TOTAL
RECOVERY

METABOLIC
CIRCADIAN
MICROBIAL
IMMUNE
MENTAL

FIVE
FITNESSES

Total Recovery splits total fitness into the five fitnesses.

Metabolic fitness. It's the resilience of the body to exertion stress, macronutrient stress, and DNA damage stress. It's strengthened by exercise, nutrition, and skincare. Its loss leads to cancer and diseases of the heart, brain, lungs, pancreas, kidneys, and liver.

Circadian fitness. It's the resilience of the circadian rhythm to disruption. It's strengthened by a consistent daily schedule for sleeping, waking, eating, and exercising. Its loss leads to Alzheimer's disease and losses in all the other fitnesses.

Microbial fitness. It's the resilience of the population of beneficial microbes in the gut and on every body surface. It's strengthened by fruit and vegetable consumption, tooth care, gum care, and skincare. Its loss leads to intestinal disorder and systemic inflammation.

Immune fitness. It's the resilience of the body to infection and inflammation. It's strengthened by an environment free of chemical toxins and pollutants, but rich in nature and biology. Its loss leads to allergy, brain inflammation, and autoimmune diseases.

Mental fitness. It's the resilience of the mind to anxiety, depression, and memory loss. It's strengthened by imagination, discipline, stress management, and the teachings of Total Recovery. Its loss leads to mood disorders and Alzheimer's disease.

The five fitnesses are interconnected. Each one supports the others, and each one depends on the others. Events in our lives tend to affect one fitness and then cascade into effects on all the others. If we neglect any one fitness, all five of them suffer.

The first two fitnesses — metabolic and circadian fitness — will be examined in more detail in later chapters of this book. The other three fitnesses will be examined in more detail in *Book Two: Biological Happiness*.

THE DUKE STUDY OF BIOLOGICAL AGE

Duke University researchers study how total fitness affects biological aging. They observe that young adults who have high total fitness at age 26 show less biological aging, less facial aging, and less mental aging when assessed again twelve years later at age 38.[1]

The Duke researchers take the study of total fitness to a new level. Their study is, quite frankly, the inspiration for biological youth and the five fitnesses. We should all be grateful for their study. Throughout this book, we'll refer back to their study with this citation.[**Duke Study**]

The Duke researchers assess the total fitness of nearly 1,000 adults at age 26 and again at age 38. They derive an estimate of the biological age of the subjects based on 18 different fitness measures listed below. They include 14 measures of metabolic fitness, one measure of microbial fitness, and three measures of immune fitness, as follows.

DUKE METABOLIC FITNESS MEASURES

Apolipoprotein B100/A1 ratio	Glycated hemoglobin
Blood pressure	High density lipoprotein
Body mass index	Lipoprotein(a)
Cardiorespiratory fitness (VO$_{2max}$)	Triglycerides
Creatinine clearance	Total cholesterol
Forced expiratory volume in one second (FEV1)	Urea nitrogen
Forced vital capacity ratio (FEV1/FVC)	Waist-hip ratio

---

1   Belsky DW, Caspi A, Houts R, Cohen HJ, Corcoran DL, Danese A, Harrington H, Israel S, Levine ME, Schaefer JD, Sugden K, Williams B, Yashin AI, Poulton R, Moffitt TE. **Quantification of biological aging in young adults.** Proc Natl Acad Sci U S A. 2015 Jul 28;112(30):E4104-10. *pubmed.gov/26150497*

DUKE MICROBIAL *and* IMMUNE FITNESS MEASURES

Periodontal disease	Leukocyte telomere length
C-reactive protein	White blood cell count

The Duke researchers estimate the rate of biological aging of the subjects over the 12-year interval, between age 26 and age 38. The subjects with high total fitness age at a rate of almost zero years per calendar year. The subjects with low total fitness age at a rate of nearly three years per calendar year.[**Duke Study**] Did you catch that? High total fitness causes people to age slowly. Low total fitness causes people to age fast!

The Duke researchers observe the following evidence for biological youth in the study subjects who maintain high total fitness. They observe less facial aging based on a facial photograph. They observe better self-reported estimates of healthiness. They observe better mental functioning. They observe better blood supply to the brain. They also observe better physical strength and mobility.[**Duke Study**]

In other words, if we increase our total fitness: we'll look younger; we'll feel younger; we'll think better; and we'll be stronger and more mobile.

The Duke researchers provide an exciting glimpse of the different aging trajectories we can choose based on our lifestyle choices and our total fitness. And keep in mind, these study subjects were chosen randomly and their lifestyles were random. The subjects were in an observational study, not a lifestyle intervention study.

But lifestyle choices don't have to be so random. We've now got TR. We've got all the answers sitting right here. Welcome to the revolution of Total Recovery, biological youth, and the five fitnesses.

THE DIMMER SWITCHES OF FITNESS

To help us visualize how total fitness depends on the five fitnesses, TR represents total fitness as a light bulb and each of the five fitnesses as a *Dimmer Switch of Fitness*. All the dimmers are wired together on the same electric circuit to control the brightness of the single light bulb of total fitness.

Full on. When EVERY dimmer is maximum, the brightness of the light bulb maximum. This state represents 100% total fitness. It represents maximum theoretical biological youth.

Full off. When any SINGLE dimmer shuts off, the light bulb shuts off. Poof! This state represents 100% frailty. It represents the state of maximum biological age and precipitates one of many possible health catastrophes we collectively call death by natural causes. Unlike maximum fitness, maximum frailty is not a theoretical state. It's completely real. It's a state all of our bodies will experience at one time or another.

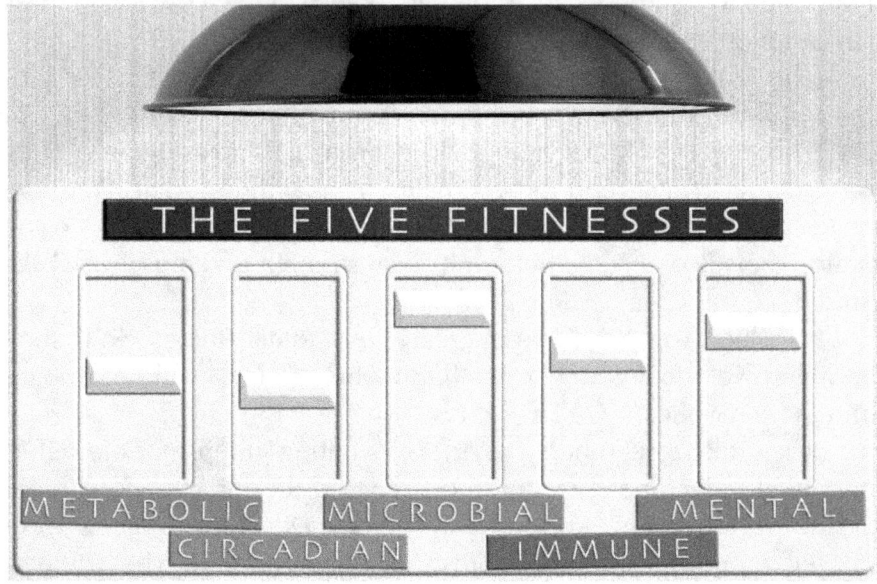

When any SINGLE dimmer shuts off, biological youth shuts off.

The mechanism of the five dimmer switches illustrates how we must strengthen EVERY ONE of the five fitnesses in order to nurture the recovery of our body's cell ecosystem and preserve our biological youth.

The mechanism of the five dimmer switches helps explain why we've always struggled to find biological youth. We've always assumed that different forms of fitness ADD up to total fitness. But they don't ADD, they MULTIPLY. They obey the property of biological synergy, which means they all must work together.[2]

As dimmers on the same electric circuit, if any single switch

---

2   Wikipedia. **Synergy.** Accessed 2016. *en.wikipedia.org/wiki/Synergy*

shuts off, it introduces a zero into the multiplication. Zero times any number is zero. Zero times four other numbers is still zero.

Multiplication is very different from addition. The sum of five numbers doesn't change very much if one of the numbers goes to zero. But the product of five numbers changes dramatically if one of them goes to zero. The whole product goes to zero. Poof!

The concept of the five dimmers of fitness changes the whole language of health advice. The math has now changed. The different parts of our health don't ADD, they MULTIPLY. To preserve biological youth, we MUST exercise, we MUST eat right, we MUST sleep right, and so on.

We've never been warned there are so many fitnesses that we MUST focus on at the same time. When we just focus on metabolic fitness, the other dimmers keep sliding down and dimming our light. And then, we throw up our hands and say,

"Aging is inevitable. It can't be stopped."

The mechanism of the five dimmers is a revolution in our understanding of human health and aging. It provides a natural strategy for sustaining our youthfulness that's never been tried before. It opens up a whole new territory for research. We don't know how far it will take us. We don't know where it may end. It's frankly exhilarating.

THE UCLA STUDY OF REVERSING ALZHEIMER'S

UCLA researchers are confirming how the five dimmers of fitness obey biological synergy with a small study to reverse Alzheimer's disease. The researchers provide a lifestyle intervention that targets 36 different lifestyle behaviors to boost all five fitnesses at once. They are testing the lifestyle intervention in a pilot study with ten patients suffering from cognitive impairment and they are observing dramatic results.[3]

The UCLA lifestyle intervention can be translated into the conceptual framework of Total Recovery and the five fitnesses as follows:

---

3   Bredesen DE. **Reversal of cognitive decline: a novel therapeutic program.** Aging (Albany NY). 2014 Sep;6(9):707-17. *pubmed.gov/ 25324467*

Metabolic Fitness

Exercise	Supplements	Test heavy metals
Up to 60 min/day	Amino acids	Cadmium
Up to 6 days/week	Enzyme cofactors	Lead
Test hormones	Healthy fats	Mercury
Estrogens	Herbs	
Stress	Minerals	
Testosterone	Polyphenols	
Thyroid	Vitamins	

Circadian Fitness

Sleep regimen	Nightly fasting	Supplements
8 hours/night	3 hrs before sleep	Melatonin
Treat sleep apnea	12 hrs/night	Tryptophan

Microbial Fitness

Diet		Dental hygiene
Low refined carbs	Prebiotics	Electric brushing
Low grains	Probiotics	Water flossing

Immune Fitness

Test inflammation markers
Albumin/globulin ratio
C-reactive protein

Mental Fitness

Stress reduction	Mental exercises
Meditation	Mental puzzles
Yoga	

The UCLA researchers are testing their lifestyle intervention with four Alzheimer's patients, ages 54, 62, 69, and 74 years, and with six mild cognitive impairment (MCI) patients, ages 49, 49, 54, 55, 66, and 68 years. Cognitive testing and MRI brain imaging both confirm a reversal of disease for all ten patients after only five to 24 months of the lifestyle intervention.[4]

---

4   Bredesen DE, Amos EC, Canick J, Ackerley M, Raji C, Fiala M, Ahdidan J. **Reversal of cognitive decline in Alzheimer's disease.** Aging (Al-

Prior to the study, the patients were struggling with keeping their jobs and with their daily lives. Once they began the lifestyle intervention, the patients noticed so much improvement, they could return to their jobs and work like they were years younger. One patient took a three-week hiatus from the lifestyle intervention and noticed an immediate decline in cognitive functioning. Upon returning to the lifestyle intervention, the patient began experiencing cognitive improvements again.

The UCLA researchers are showing how lifestyle intervention can be a viable therapy for Alzheimer's disease, which is estimated to be the number three killer behind cardiovascular disease and cancer.[5] With its current trend of increasing prevalence, Alzheimer's disease could singlehandedly bankrupt the U.S. Medicare system. Women are now more likely to die from Alzheimer's disease than breast cancer.[6]

We're entering an exciting time for lifestyle intervention research. The UCLA researchers are demonstrating that a total fitness-based lifestyle intervention is not only practical, it effectively reverses the biological age of our brains. Their work is an inspiration for health and fitness advocates and is frankly the inspiration for the Five Dimmers of Fitness. We should all be grateful for the work of the UCLA researchers.

THE **THEORY** OF **BIOLOGICAL YOUTH**

We're used to thinking about our age in calendar years. When we think about biological age, we tend to think about it in calendar years too. Total Recovery defines biological age 20 as the point when we have 100% fitness and biological age 80 when we have 100% frailty. Each of us is on our own aging trajectory and will reach biological age 80 at a different calendar age. Some of us may reach it at calendar age 50, while some of us may reach it at calen-

bany NY). 2016 Jun;8(6):1250-8. *pubmed.gov/27294343*

5   James BD, Leurgans SE, Hebert LE, Scherr PA, Yaffe K, Bennett DA. **Contribution of Alzheimer disease to mortality in the United States.** Neurology. 2014 Mar 25;82(12):1045-50. *pubmed.gov/24598707*

6   Alzheimer's Association. **2014 Alzheimer's disease facts and figures.** Alzheimers Dement. 2014 Mar;10(2):e47-92. *pubmed.gov/24818261*

dar age 110.

Biological youth is the complete opposite of biological age, so we need a new kind of math to represent it. For all the math lovers out there, Total Recovery presents to you the Theory of Biological Youth as a series of mathematical equations. Here we go.

Biological youth — or youthfulness — is represented as a percentage. It can then be related mathematically to total fitness when both are in the form of percentages.

%Youthfulness = %Fitness

Biological age — or agedness — can also be represented as a percentage in order to compare it to total frailty.

%Agedness = %Frailty

Youthfulness and fitness are like thinking of a glass as half FULL. Agedness and frailty are like thinking of a glass as half EMPTY. Between biological age 20 (100% fitness) and 80 (100% frailty), our bodies are partly FIT and partly FRAIL as follows:

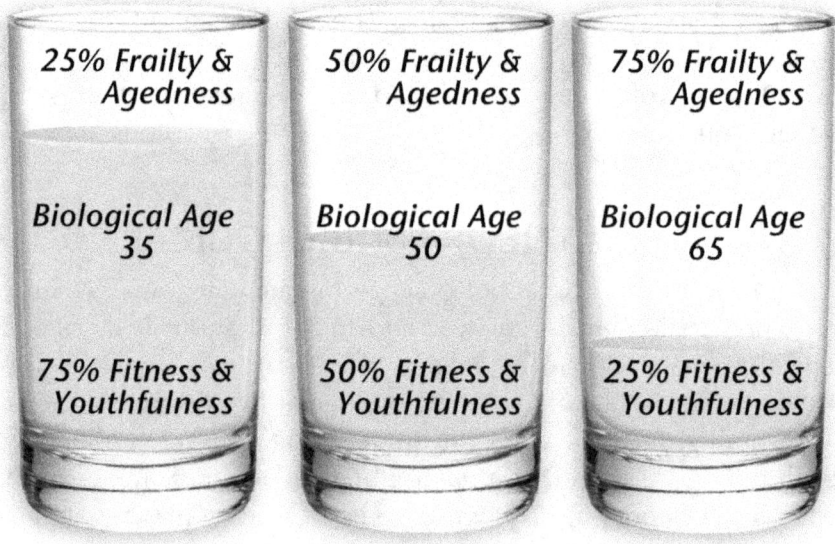

%Frailty + %Fitness = 100%

%Agedness + %Youthfulness = 100%

The theory of biological youth encourages us to strengthen our total fitness, giving us direct control over the youthfulness of our bodies. Because total fitness is the most fundamental quantity researchers can measure, TR derives all the other quantities from total fitness as follows:

%Youthfulness = %Fitness

%Frailty = 100% − %Fitness

%Agedness = 100% − %Fitness

As total fitness approaches 100%, youthfulness approaches 100%. Agedness and total frailty approach 0%. 100% total fitness is the theoretical maximum fitness that can be attained by a young adult. We can't get any more fit than our theoretical maximum in young adulthood.

As total fitness approaches 0%, youthfulness approaches 0%. Agedness and total frailty approach 100%. 100% total frailty is equivalent to the moment of death by natural causes. We can't get any more frail than at the point of multiple organ failure.

Total fitness can be maintained naturally. It does not require pharmaceuticals, surgery, or high-tech stem cell therapy. It puts the ball back in our court and lets us hold on to it as long as possible.

When we NURTURE total fitness, we nurture youthfulness.

When we NEGLECT total fitness, we nurture frailty and agedness.

Biological youth is remarkably elegant. It's like an instruction manual for managing the ecosystem of cells in our bodies. It gives us all the directions we need.

People complain that youth is wasted on the young and that aging is not for sissies. Biological youth changes all that.

THE **TRADITIONAL THEORY** OF **AGING**

The traditional theory of aging is that damage accumulates in the body.[7] This theory causes us to dwell on the structural components in our bodies rather than on our cell ecosystem. This theory guides us in the wrong direction for the following reasons:

Static vs. dynamic. The damage concept makes us think of our body parts as static objects that wear out like the parts of a building. But our body parts are dynamic, not static. Our body uses stem cells

---

7   Wikipedia. **Aging.** Accessed 2016. *en.wikipedia.org/wiki/Ageing*

to replace old cells.[8] When we preserve the fitness of our cell ecosystem, we preserve our population of stem cells and we allow our body parts to heal themselves.

Tissue turnover. The damage concept fails to recognize the constant turnover of tissue as cells are removed and replaced. It overlooks how most tissues completely replace themselves regularly. The heart, for example, effectively replaces itself every eight years.[9] The skeleton effectively replaces itself every 12 years.[**10**] Fat tissue effectively replaces itself every 16 years.[**11**]

Adaptation to use. The damage concept fails to consider how many of the changes we observe with age are simply the result of the long-term remodeling our bodies undergo to ADAPT to how we USE them. Our bodies remodel our tissues to match how we use our tissues. Our bodies shed muscle and bone when we don't use them. Our bodies accumulate fat to store the excess calories we eat.

Youthful features. Young adults tend to have a narrow range of facial and body features. The older we get, the more our bodies remodel themselves to adapt to our unique lifestyle habits. Consequently, older adults have a wider spectrum of facial and body features. Think of when you walk behind someone you assume is young. When they turn around, you see their face, and you're surprised to see how much older they are. It's because their body features fit within the narrow range of features that we associate with a young body. Much of the changes we observe in older adult bodies

---

8   Wikipedia. **Stem cell.** Accessed 2016. *en.wikipedia.org/wiki/Stem_cell*

9   Kajstura J, Gurusamy N, Ogórek B, Goichberg P, Clavo-Rondon C, Hosoda T, D'Amario D, Bardelli S, Beltrami AP, Cesselli D, Bussani R, del Monte F, Quaini F, Rota M, Beltrami CA, Buchholz BA, Leri A, Anversa P. **Myocyte turnover in the aging human heart.** Circ Res. 2010 Nov 26;107(11):1374-86. *pubmed.gov/21088285*

10   Manolagas SC. **Birth and death of bone cells: basic regulatory mechanisms and implications for the pathogenesis and treatment of osteoporosis.** Endocr Rev. 2000 Apr;21(2):115-37. *pubmed.gov/10782361*

11   Spalding KL, Arner E, Westermark PO, Bernard S, Buchholz BA, Bergmann O, Blomqvist L, Hoffstedt J, Näslund E, Britton T, Concha H, Hassan M, Rydén M, Frisén J, Arner P. **Dynamics of fat cell turnover in humans.** Nature. 2008 Jun 5;453(7196):783-7. *pubmed.gov/18454136*

can be reversed with a lifestyle intervention because the changes aren't permanent damage but simply the result of remodeling.

Hunchback. Consider how some people develop a hunchback. It is technically called kyphosis, a Greek word for hump.[12] The most common form is called postural kyphosis and is attributed to persistent slouching. It is corrected with postural therapy. The rounded back appears damaged, but most of the time, it's not damaged. The rounded back has simply remodeled itself to accommodate years of slouching. With physical therapy, the rounded back returns to normal as its use returns to normal.

Wearing a cast. Consider how our muscles shrink when we wear a cast. It is technically called atrophy, a Greek word for undernourished.[13] When the cast comes off, the arm or leg looks shriveled — to the point it appears almost comical. But within weeks of use, the muscle rebuilds back to normal. Bang! The shriveled muscle isn't damaged. It's just remodeled to fit our lack of use. Its size returns to normal as its use returns to normal.

Death by natural causes. The damage concept makes us think our body will get old and die when it has accumulated a critical amount of damage. In reality, our bodies have redundant mechanisms of body system regulation to compensate for deficiencies in any one system.[14] With greater fitness, a body becomes more resilient to damage. For instance, people with greater physical strength are more likely to recover from traumatic injury.[15] In reality, death is caused by an **insufficiency of fitness** to accommodate an insult rather than by any particular accumulation of damage.

The damage theory of aging has unintended consequences. It makes us think our aging is out of our control. We tell ourselves there's nothing we can do about it. The damage theory gives us an

---

12   Wikipedia. **Kyphosis.** Accessed 2016. *en.wikipedia.org/wiki/Kyphosis*

13   Wikipedia. **Muscle atrophy.** Accessed 2016. *en.wikipedia.org/wiki/Muscle_atrophy*

14   Wikipedia. **Homeostasis.** Accessed 2016. *en.wikipedia.org/wiki/Homeostasis*

15   Lee JJ, Waak K, Grosse-Sundrup M, Xue F, Lee J, Chipman D, Ryan C, Bittner EA, Schmidt U, Eikermann M. **Global muscle strength but not grip strength predicts mortality and length of stay in a general population in a surgical intensive care unit.** Phys Ther. 2012 Dec; 92(12):1546-55. *pubmed.gov/22976446*

excuse for not trying. We say to ourselves,

"When my body was young, it could do those things. But now that it's old, it can't do them anymore."

The damage theory of aging becomes a white lie we tell ourselves. We repeat it to ourselves over and over, so we don't feel so bad about what we've done to our bodies.

The damage theory of aging causes us to think in a magical fashion about high-tech medicine and alternative treatments. We think there's a cure for our damage, and we think we can find someone who will give it to us. Likely, we end up in our doctor's office. Likely, we end up discussing how to remove the damage from our bodies.

FITNESS and FRAILTY

In TR, we define biological youth as total fitness of the body. And in TR, we consider all perspectives. We use fitness and youthfulness. And we use frailty and agedness. Each provides a different perspective. Each has its advantages. They're all needed to better describe the changes in the body over time.

Total fitness has the advantage of being positively motivating. It encourages us to reflect on our five fitnesses and how they have changed since we were a young adult. We can assess each of the fitnesses by its strength and its resilience to stress.

To understand resilience to stress, consider metabolic fitness. When it's high, the body can sprint at a high speed during an emergency. When it's low, the same sprint would cause lung pain, heart pain, and potentially a heart attack.

- 100% total fitness means each of the five fitnesses provides us 100% resiliency to every stress in normal life.
- 0% total fitness means at least one of the five fitnesses has become 100% vulnerable to any minuscule stress — complete frailty.

Total fitness gives us the big picture so we can understand how every one of the five fitnesses is essential. It treats the body as a dynamic system with parts that can heal and repair when used properly. It trains us to keep all parts working and functioning together.

Fitness motivates us to do the right thing. It motivates us to exercise our bodies and our minds. We might end up at the gym, on a hike, in the fresh produce section, or at the library.

In TR, we define biological age as total frailty of the body. We use the concept of frailty, instead of accumulated damage, because it better describes how a dynamic system is vulnerable to failure when placed under stress. Frailty is the mirror image of fitness.

People often represent biological age, or agedness, in units of years because it typically correlates with calendar age. In TR, we define the beginning of adulthood as biological age 20, which typically corresponds to calendar age 20. We define the end of adulthood, or death by natural causes, as biological age 80, which typically corresponds to calendar age 80, on average, for the population of U.S. adults.

For some adults, death by natural causes, or biological age 80, arrives as early as calendar age 50, giving them only 30 years of adulthood. For many adults, biological age 80 corresponds to calendar age 80, giving them 60 years of adulthood. For some rare adults, biological age 80 corresponds to calendar age 110, giving them 90 years of adulthood.

Based on these definitions of agedness, we can now put everything together. We can consider how declining fitness and increasing frailty relate to major health risks. These trends in health risk are summarized below in the *Fitness and Frailty Chart*.

FITNESS AND FRAILTY CHART

Fitness	Frailty	Biological Age	Calendar Age	Main Risks
100%	0%	20	20	Accidents
75%	25%	35	/ \	—
50%	50%	50	35 - 65	Disorders
25%	75%	65	/ \	Diseases
0%	100%	80	50 — 110	Death

The *Fitness and Frailty Chart* is a preliminary sketch of the trends. We'll add more details throughout the series of Total Recovery books. We'll also need the help of researchers — to study these concepts, kick them around, test them out, and start using them.

THE **TOTAL FITNESS EXAM**

Total Recovery provides a conceptual framework for a future in which we could quantify our total fitness and our biological youth. Imagine a day when we have the opportunity to request a Total Fitness Exam from our personal doctors. It would be like an annual physical exam, plus the Duke Study, plus the UCLA Study, and even more. It would be over-the-top thorough.

Such an exam may entail the following steps:

- We'd set aside a whole day for the exam.
- We'd fill out an electronic survey beforehand to provide information about our lifestyle and our food intake over the last few days.
- We'd drink a cocktail of diagnostic solutions to assess intestine and kidney function.
- We'd give saliva, urine, stool, and blood samples.
- We'd undergo a treadmill test, cardiorespiratory exam, periodontal exam, and dermatology exam.
- We'd spend the night in a sleep lab to assess circadian fitness.

When all the samples from the Total Fitness Exam are analyzed and reviewed by a qualified professional, a Total Fitness Report would be generated and provided to us and our doctors. It might have a fitness summary that looks like one of the examples below.

The summary might report total fitness as a percentage and each of the five fitnesses as percentages and colored bars.

Our doctors may go over the full report and highlight key areas to work on. They may include their own observations about our unique health status that go beyond the Total Fitness Report. They may refer us to a physical therapist, dietitian, or dermatologist to provide us more guidance.

The Total Fitness Exam would be so THOROUGH it would intimidate most people. But keep in mind, as we age, we have to endure uncomfortable screening tests such as colonoscopies, pap smears, and mammograms. These screening tests simply report whether we are at a low, moderate, or heightened risk of cancer.

The Total Fitness Exam would be more time-consuming, but it would give us a result that would be far more motivating. It's an actual number that shows us how much fitness and how much biological youth we've still got left in us. With a read-out in hand, we can start modifying our lifestyle and see how much better we can do the next time.

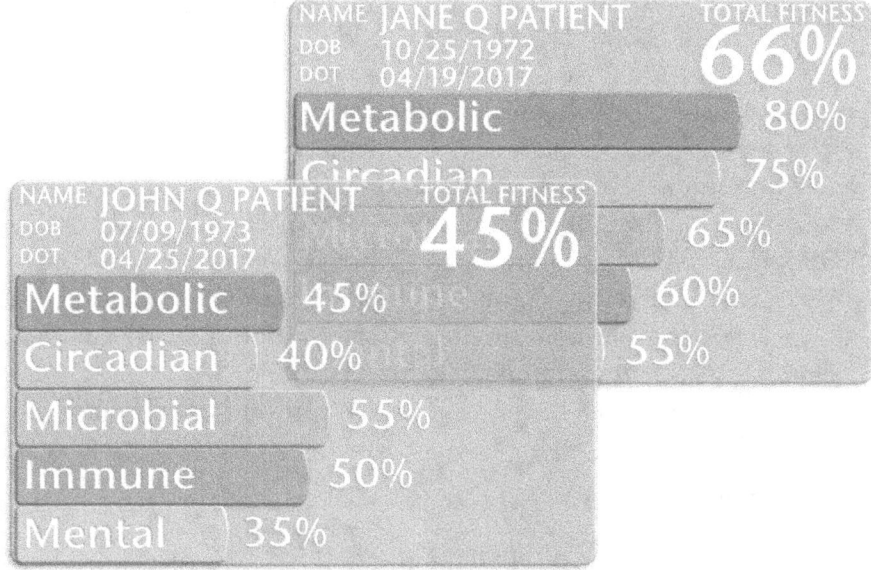

Summary of the Total Fitness Report

In time, health insurance companies may choose to cover the cost completely as an incentive to subscribers. The Exam may motivate us to make lifestyle changes, see our fitness scores improve, and reduce our risks of disease and death.

The Total Fitness Report may become a win-win for everyone involved in health care.

CHAPTER ONE REVIEW

Biological youth. Also known as youthfulness, biological youth is defined as the total fitness of the body. Fitness represents resilience to every stress in normal life. Fitness is sustained by a healthy lifestyle and a healthy environment.

Fitness and youthfulness have a theoretical MAXIMUM in early adulthood, around age 20. Fitness and youthfulness have a theoretical MINIMUM at the moment of death by natural causes.

Biological age. Also known as agedness, biological age is defined as the total frailty of the body. Frailty represents vulnerability to any stress in normal life. Frailty is promoted by an unhealthy lifestyle and an unhealthy environment.

Youthfulness, agedness, and frailty can be derived from fitness as follows.

%Youthfulness = %Fitness

%Frailty = 100% − %Fitness

%Agedness = 100% − %Fitness

As fitness declines, youthfulness declines, frailty increases, and agedness increases. Frailty and biological age are suppressed when fitness is sustained. They increase when fitness is neglected.

Frailty and biological age have a theoretical minimum in early adulthood, around age 20. They have a theoretical maximum at the moment of death by natural causes.

Total fitness. It is computed by MULTIPLYING together the five fitnesses. Like a lightbulb connected to a panel of five dimmer switches, total fitness fails when ANY of the five fitnesses fail. Total frailty is the mirror image of total fitness.

Metabolic fitness. It is the resilience of the body to exertion, nutrient, and DNA damage stress. It is fostered by prudent exercise, nutrition, and skincare. Metabolic frailty associates with cancer, frailty syndrome, and loss of organ function.

Circadian fitness. It is the resilience of circadian rhythm to disruption. It is fostered by adherence to a consistent rhythm for sleeping, waking, eating, and exercising. Circadian frailty associates with Alzheimer's disease, mental frailty, and metabolic frailty.

Microbial fitness. It is the resilience of the population of beneficial microbes in the gut and on every body surface. It is fostered by prudent nutrition, tooth care, gum care, and skincare.

Immune fitness. It is the resilience of the body to infection and inflammation. It is fostered by an environment free of chemical toxins and pollutants, but rich in nature and biology. It is particularly inter-connected with the four other fitnesses.

Mental fitness. It is the resilience of the mind to anxiety, depression, impulsivity, and indulgence. It is strengthened by imagination, discipline, stress management, and the teachings of Total Recovery.

UCLA Study of Reversing Alzheimer's. UCLA researchers report on a successful pilot study of a lifestyle intervention with ten cognitive impairment patients. The 36-point lifestyle intervention addresses all five fitnesses in a way that is consistent with their synergistic relationship and the multiplicative contribution of each *Dimmer Switch of Fitness* to the brightness of total fitness.

Total fitness exam. It would be a comprehensive physical exam of the five fitnesses. The exam would guide us as to how to adjust our lifestyle to sustain our youthfulness as long as possible.

CHAPTER ONE IMAGINE

The Total Fitness Exam would be a major commitment of time, unlike any other medical exam. The idea of spending an entire day and night in a clinical laboratory would overwhelm most of us. We would need the Exam offered to us in different formats to better suit our unique schedules and commitments.

In the distant future, wearable devices may play a role in the Exam. People inspired by the Quantified Self movement would want to collect this kind of data with their fitness trackers every day. Perhaps in the future, device manufacturers will team up with researchers to make trackers for all of the five fitnesses. Researchers may need to develop in-home saliva, blood, urine, and stool test kits.

In the nearer future, health resorts may play a role in the Exam. Such a resort offering the Exam may be called a Total Fitness Resort. The resort would be staffed with technicians and researchers. It wouldn't have any phony baloney, just lots of testing equipment and specimen collection facilities.

We might enjoy traveling to such a destination, like it's a vacation. Our insurance might cover the Exam, but we might pay to stay longer, just like a real resort. We might sign up for fitness classes, cooking classes, skincare classes, sleep coaching, mindfulness training, and stress management. Total Recovery could even help out with the workshops and classes. Guests might enjoy health classes taught with the playfulness and the seriousness of TR.

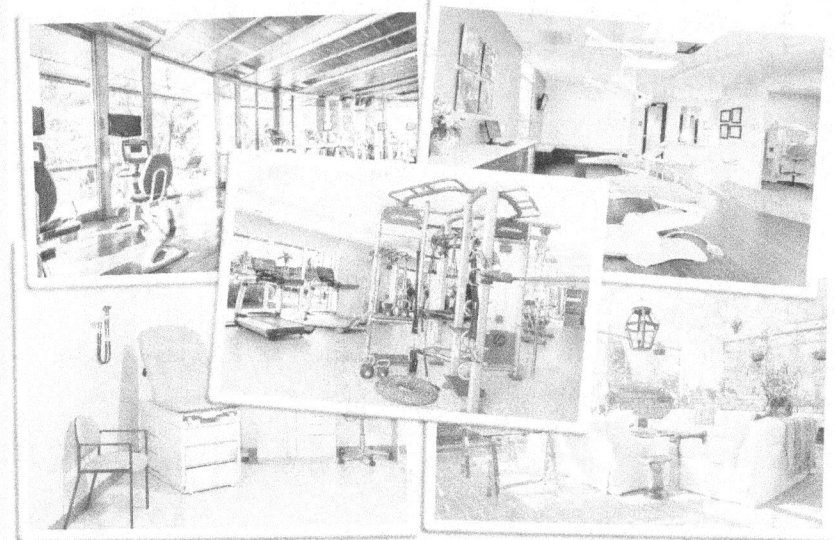

The Total Fitness Exam could be provided at a Total Fitness Resort.

Every guest at the Total Fitness RESORT would receive a Total Fitness REPORT. It's kind of catchy.

The Total Fitness Exam has the potential to influence the future of health care. Imagine fewer hospitals and more fitness resorts. Imagine decreased health care expenses for frailty and agedness and increased health care resources available for fitness and biological youth.

Future health care will be less expensive and more effective. Say hello to total fitness and biological youth.

ZOMBIE BEHAVIORS

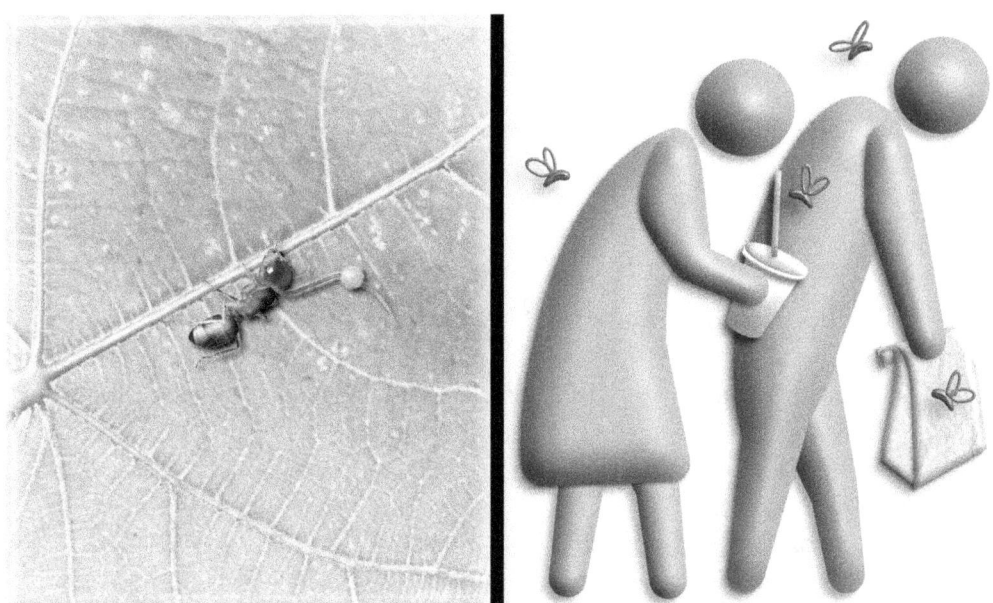

Our zombie behaviors undermine our long-term health.

With every new advance in health research, the gap widens between what we KNOW we should do and what we ACTUALLY do. We know we should exercise more, but we don't. We know we should eat more vegetables, but we don't. Do you ever wonder why we know so much, and yet we continue to engage in behaviors that undermine our long-term health?

Say hello to zombie behaviors. They're the erratic behaviors of zombie insects in nature whose decision-making has been subverted by parasites. It turns out we have zombie behaviors too. Our zombie behaviors are encouraged by companies selling us things, by voices in the media, by our friends, and by our family members. We must take control of our zombie behaviors before we can ACTUALLY do what we KNOW we should do.

In this chapter, we examine the following topics:

BIOLOGICAL ZOMBIES in NATURE

Hollywood zombies are so entrenched in our culture, it's easy to overlook the real-life biological zombies found in nature. Zombie ants, zombie caterpillars, and zombie grasshoppers have been identified by scientists. These creatures help us understand how zombie behaviors occur naturally whenever decision-making is subverted by outside forces.

Zombie ants. Carpenter ants infected with a zombie fungus called *Cordyceps* can be found in tropical rain forests. Carpenter ants live in colonies high in the trees in the rain forest canopy. When an ant becomes infected with *Cordyceps*, it experiences muscle seizures and falls from the tree branches down to the forest floor where the humidity better suits *Cordyceps*.[16]

On the forest floor, the carpenter ant transforms into a biological zombie and wanders erratically while awaiting instructions from *Cordyceps*. At precisely noon-time, when the sun is highest, *Cordyceps* assumes full control over the brain of the ant.

The zombie ant abruptly stops walking, climbs up a plant, and searches for a leaf in a location carefully selected by *Cordyceps*. The leaf must be exactly 10 inches from the ground on the north-facing side of the plant where the temperature and humidity are ideal for *Cordyceps* to mature.[17]

---

16   Wikipedia. **Ophiocordyceps unilateralis.** Accessed 2016. *en. wikipedia.org/wiki/Ophiocordyceps_unilateralis*

17   Hughes DP, Andersen SB, Hywel-Jones NL, Himaman W, Billen J, Boomsma JJ. **Behavioral mechanisms and morphological symptoms**

The zombie ant attaches its mandible to a major vein on the underside of the leaf. It applies so much force with its mandible that it forms a characteristic indentation on the leaf. The ant remains in a death grip, dangling under the leaf, away from its colony, all by itself.

Within a week, *Cordyceps* destroys the brain and internal tissues of the ant. It kills the ant while the ant remains attached in its death grip and dangles under the leaf. It grows a fruiting body out through the head of the ant. Within another week, *Cordyceps* completes its life cycle and releases infectious spores from the fruiting body.

The zombie ant follows its instructions alone, but it has plenty of company. Naturalists count up to 30 zombie ants in one square meter of forest floor. Naturalists also observe the characteristic death grip indentations on fossilized leaves that date back nearly 50 million years.

Zombie caterpillars. In Brazil, caterpillars are enslaved by parasitic wasps. When a zombie caterpillar becomes enslaved, it carries the wasp's eggs until the eggs hatch. It covers the larvae with silk and guards them. The zombie caterpillar fights off approaching predators by swinging its head wildly.[18]

A caterpillar normally builds a chrysalis to become a butterfly or moth. A caterpillar dreams of flying. But a zombie caterpillar gives up that dream. It guards the wasp larvae, swinging its head at predators, until it dies of starvation.

Zombie grasshoppers. Parasitic worms enslaves grasshoppers. When a zombie grasshopper becomes enslaved, it carries the worm's eggs until they hatch, and it deposits the larvae into water. [19] The grasshopper doesn't know how to swim. It doesn't like wa-

of zombie ants dying from fungal infection. BMC Ecol. 2011 May 9;11:13. *pubmed.gov/21554670*

18   Grosman AH, Janssen A, de Brito EF, Cordeiro EG, Colares F, Fonseca JO, Lima ER, Pallini A, Sabelis MW. **Parasitoid increases survival of its pupae by inducing hosts to fight predators.** PLoS One. 2008 Jun 4;3(6):e2276. *pubmed.gov/18523578*

19   Ponton F, Otálora-Luna F, Lefèvre T, Guerin PM, Lebarbenchon C, Duneau D, Biron DG, Thomas F. **Water-seeking behavior in worm-infected crickets and reversibility of parasitic manipulation.** Behav Ecol. 2011 Mar;22(2):392-400. *pubmed.gov/22476265*

ter. Yet the zombie grasshopper risks drowning to make sure the worm larvae are deposited safely back into water.

Zombie ants, caterpillars, and grasshoppers all engage in behaviors that harm their health and benefit a parasite. Biological zombies are real. They are part of nature. They are around us right now. And they have been for millions of years.

OUR ZOMBIE BEHAVIORS

We inherit the concept of the human zombie from enslaved West Africans brought to Haiti during the era of European colonialism. In Haitian folklore, a zombie is an undead person enslaved by a sorcerer. Scholars suggest the zombie is a cultural metaphor for Haiti's struggles with slavery.[20]

The biological zombie and the Haitian zombie provide a unique way to think about the difficulty we have sticking with healthy behaviors. We can imagine how our unhealthy behaviors are zombie behaviors. And, we can imagine how they are caused by zombie viruses — or bad ideas — spread to us by advertisers, media, family, and friends.

Zombie behaviors are quite deadly. We're facing an epidemic of diseases that health professionals classify as **non-communicable diseases** (**NCDs**). NCDs includes diabetes, cardiovascular disease, cancer, Alzheimer's disease, lung disease, and autoimmune disease. These diseases are not transmitted by infectious agents between people. They're caused by our behaviors and our exposure to pollution.[21]

NCDs are the leading cause of death around the world. In 2012, 38 million deaths were caused by NCDs, which is 68% of all deaths, up from 60% in 2000. NCDs are not necessarily old person diseases; half of all NCD deaths occur to people under age 70. NCDs are increasing because of our changing lifestyles and our increasing exposure to pollution.

Air pollution is the most immediate environmental problem contributing to NCDs. It causes inflammation in the lungs, leading

---

20   Wikipedia. **Zombie.** Accessed 2016. *en.wikipedia.org/wiki/Zombie*

21   Wikipedia. **Non-communicable disease.** Accessed 2016.   *en.wikipedia.org/wiki/Non-communicable_disease*

to asthma, bronchitis, emphysema, and lung cancer. It causes inflammation in the heart and blood vessels, leading to high blood pressure, heart attacks, and stroke. It even causes inflammation in the brain, leading to memory impairment, behavior disorder, and autism disorders. Air pollution is estimated to kill seven million people every year, which is nearly 20% of the 38 million deaths from NCDs. In the Los Angeles area, air pollution is estimated to kill more people than traffic collisions.[22]

OUR ZOMBIE VIRUSES

We rarely question beliefs and behaviors that we perceive to be mainstream. We assume that if others share our mainstream beliefs and behaviors, then everything must be fine. We don't realize the extent to which marketers shape mainstream beliefs through advertising in a fashion that can be likened to the transmission of zombie viruses.

Viral marketing. Marketing agencies work to create increasingly potent zombie viruses to increase the sales and consumption of their products. Marketers use the term viral marketing to describe how an advertisement reaches a "susceptible" user and "infects" that user. When an infected user shares the advertisement and "infects" another susceptible user, the number of infected users grows like an epidemic.[23] These concepts from viral marketing take on new meaning once we understand zombie behaviors and viruses.

Internet marketing. The internet connects us to so much health information, we should all be health geniuses by now. But since we don't like to pay for information on the internet, we're stuck with high-pressure internet marketing on every page. Even the most reputable web sites serve us click-bait such as "The amazing skinny pill that doctors hate," or "The three foods you should NEVER eat."[24] Internet marketing seems to increasingly breed health misinformation and zombie viruses in order to capture our fleeting attention.

---

22 Wikipedia. **Air pollution.** Accessed 2016. *en.wikipedia.org/wiki/Air_pollution*

23 Wikipedia. **Viral marketing.** Accessed 2016. *en.wikipedia.org/wiki/Viral_marketing*

24 Wikipedia. **Clickbait.** Accessed 2016. *en.wikipedia.org/wiki/Clickbait*

Neuromarketing. The most troubling development in marketing is the use of medical brain imaging to study how the brains of test subjects respond to advertising messages. Marketers use the term neuromarketing to describe their use of medical devices such as magnetic resonance imaging (MRI), electroencephalography (EEG), steady state topography (SST), heart monitors, respiratory monitors, and skin moisture sensors.[25] Such devices were intended for the evaluation of brain health, not for the subversion of our mindfulness and our decision making.

Marketers use neuromarketing to target responses in specific regions of our brains with their advertising. They may develop such effective responses in our brains that we will need to re-evaluate our concepts of marketing influence, personal decision making, zombie viruses, and zombie behaviors.

A CALL FOR ZOMBIE BEHAVIOR RESEARCH

Total Recovery, or TR, is designed in part to help researchers address our looming crises of non-communicable disease and environmental pollution. To this end, TR proposes the concepts of zombie behaviors and zombie viruses to help us get to the root cause of our looming crises.

Here are the key concepts.

Biological zombies. They're creatures in nature controlled by parasites. Biological zombies adopt behaviors that undermine their health while providing benefit to the parasites. Biological zombies are typically insects. Zombie parasites are typically fungi, insects, or worms. The biological zombie provides a scientific precedent for how free will is manipulated in the animal and plant kingdoms.

Zombie behaviors. They're human behaviors that undermine our long-term health or the health of our environment. They're often encouraged by product marketing. Researchers could create an inventory of the most common zombie behaviors that increase our risk for non-communicable diseases. They could analyze the extent to which these behaviors are shaped by transmissible beliefs generated by a third party.

---

25   Wikipedia. **Neuromarketing.** Accessed 2016. *en.wikipedia.org/wiki/Neuromarketing*

Psychologists commonly use these kinds of behavior inventories to assess a variety of conditions such as mood disorders.[26] Zombie behaviors provides a new way for public health researchers to study health promotion and disease prevention.[27]

*Recovery behavior*s. They're the opposite of zombie behaviors. They're the behaviors that help us recover our health and recover the health of our environment.

*Zombie virus*es. They're transmissible beliefs often associated with product marketing that promote zombie behaviors. They're transmitted by advertisers, broadcast media, social media, and infected people. They're generally more virulent than beliefs that promote recovery behaviors.

Researchers could identify the most important zombie viruses based on the behaviors they induce and how much these behaviors erode our health and erode the environment. They could develop interventions to neutralize key zombie viruses. They could scientifically validate whether these interventions are effective at reducing zombie behaviors.

ZOMBIE BEHAVIORS AND MINDFULNESS

Total Recovery is primarily designed to increase our mindfulness and inspire us to adopt recovery behaviors — behaviors that are good for our health AND good for the environment. TR encourages us to PLAYFULLY consider how our zombie behaviors add up to making us act like zombies. This next part of TR is purely to help us with mindfulness and motivation.

Here are three prototypical zombie roles we can use to help us visualize our relative balance of zombie behaviors and recovery behaviors.

Normal zombies. They represent typical members of Western society. They understand the importance of mindfulness, health, and the environment, yet they engage in zombie behaviors. They embrace the motto, "Everything in moderation," which they use to

---

26   Wikipedia. **General Behavior Inventory.** Accessed 2016. *en.wikipedia.org/wiki/General_Behavior_Inventory*

27   Wikipedia. **Public health.** Accessed 2016. *en.wikipedia.org/wiki/Public_health*

rationalize their zombie behaviors. Normal zombies contribute to the looming crises of non-communicable disease and environmental pollution facing our society.

Recovering zombies. They represent followers of Total Recovery. They embrace the motto, "Preserve our environment, preserve our health." Recovering zombies seek mindfulness. They engage in mostly recovery behaviors and few zombie behaviors. They contribute little to the looming crises of non-communicable disease and environmental pollution.

Full-throttle zombies. They represent pleasure seekers and thrill seekers in Western society. They embrace the motto, "You only live once." Full-throttle zombies tend not to seek mindfulness. They engage in few recovery behaviors and mostly zombie behaviors. They disproportionately contribute to the looming crises of non-communicable disease and environmental pollution.

THE JOURNEY TO RECOVERY

In Total Recovery, we embark on a journey to recovery. We move away from the Western lifestyle and toward a recovery lifestyle. This journey is really a journey inside the mind.

Our minds are vulnerable to the incessant marketing of food, drink, entertainment. Our minds become filled with zombie viruses. We must seek mindfulness and the recovery from the indulgent beliefs of the Western lifestyle before we can nurture the recovery in our bodies.

The journey to recovery borrows concepts from the recovery model used to treat substance addictions and mental disorders.[28] Because TR utilizes satire, the journey to recovery is something like a tribute to — and a parody of — the twelve-step program for recovery. The Western lifestyle is full of addictive foods, beverages, leisure, and entertainment. It'll take both seriousness and humor to tackle these addictions.

This book won't be like any self-help book you've ever seen. It'll feel like we are stacking up a science book, an imagination book, a humor book, and a zombie book. And it'll feel like we're

---

28   Wikipedia. **Recovery approach.** Accessed 2016. *en.wikipedia.org/ wiki/Recovery_approach*

forcing them all through a wood chipper. Whatever's left may not be pretty, but it's a lot more interesting.

This book provides a preview of the journey ahead. It leads us on a tour through the science of youthfulness and the strategies of Total Recovery. Later books will continue the journey deeper into the science and strategies of TR.

The entire *Total Recovery Series* is attempting to do something that no other health series has ever done. Together, we will experience something truly historic, revolutionary, bizarre, and spectacular. TR opens the zombie mind, surgically removes unhealthy ideas, and implants healthy concepts. It's surprisingly effective at opening the mind.

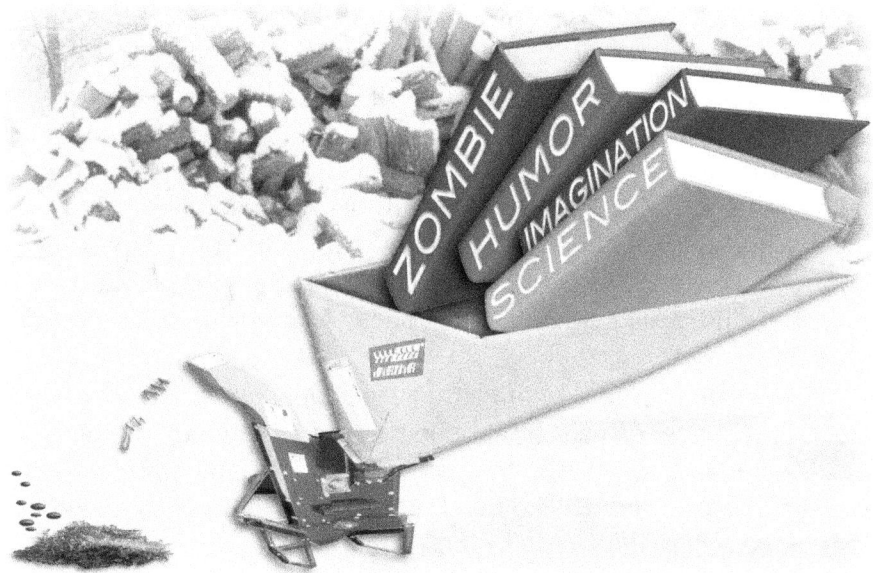

Whatever's left may not be pretty ...

TR walks freely between the worlds of sheer playfulness and utter seriousness. It helps us see the humor in our cherished health dogma and our cherished leisure culture. It sets us up to have a lot of fun together.

ENSURING A SUCCESSFUL JOURNEY

Books in the *Total Recovery Series* will stretch your powers of imagination. To prevent your head from aching, you'll need to step away periodically, close your eyes, focus on mindfulness, and just process the imagery.

Imagination. Many of our health problems exist because of our lack of imagination. It's missing at every level of our health care system. Health experts lack imagination when they lecture us with health facts. We lack imagination ourselves when we tune out what we don't want to hear. We are glutted in health INFORMATION, but we're starved of health IMAGINATION. *(Zombies tend to struggle with imagination.)*

Motivation. This book is designed for all of us zombies. It nourishes our imagination to help us visualize what our zombie behaviors are doing to us and to our environment. It nourishes our sense of humor to help us laugh at ourselves. Imagination and humor are powerful motivators. They make the choice between zombie behaviors and recovery behaviors a no-brainer. *(Zombies do better with no-brainers.)*

Learning. This book will build on concepts quickly. To keep up with the flow of new concepts, you'll need to take breaks and read the background material provided by the links to Wikipedia and PubMed. This book cannot explain all the background material. If it did, it would be a million pages long. *(Zombies tend not to read such long books.)*

Unlearning. And don't freak out if it's been forever since you've taken a science class. Our understanding of human biology has changed so much recently that you might have an advantage. You won't have to UNLEARN so much OLD science. *(Zombies tend not to remove things stuck in their brains.)*

THE FULL-THROTTLE ZOMBIE

It's important to acknowledge there are zombies among us who will never want to begin a journey to recovery.

For a normal zombie, health and the environment are important. For a recovering zombie, health and the environment are the MOST important things. But for a full-throttle zombie, other things are more important — and that's just fine.

They get tremendous satisfaction from zombie behaviors. They may explore the limits of unhealthiness or environmental unfriendliness like it's a form of artistic expression or a religious pilgrimage to be bad. We refer to them as full-throttle zombies, and it's meant with affection, not disrespect.

The TR series will steer away from trash talk about people based on their health and environmental choices. When TR uses phrases such as "unhealthy behavior," "zombie behavior," "bad for health," or "bad for the environment," it simply refers to effects on health and the environment. TR isn't judging the person, their morality, their ethics, or their value to society.

In fact, we should consider why the full-throttle zombie is quite VALUABLE to society. We should consider the reasons a full-throttle zombie should NOT start a journey to recovery.

First, medical researchers need the full-throttle zombie. Researchers need data from people with healthy lifestyles AND unhealthy lifestyles. The full-throttle zombie is the research subject who willingly eats all the bad food and takes all the bad drugs and shows us what the human body can withstand.

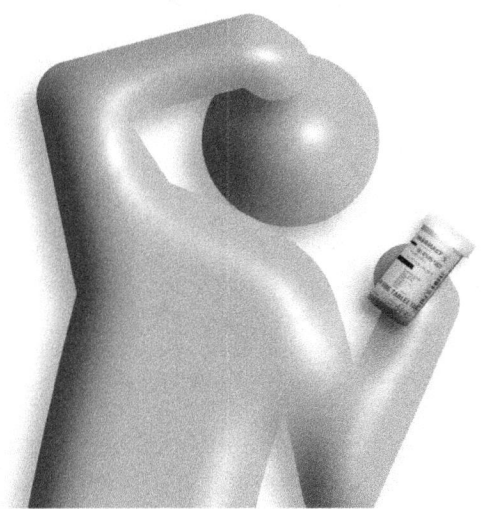

Someone who takes all the bad drugs.

Medical researchers need this kind of data. And the more data the better. They need the full-throttle zombie to keep doing what they do best. To medical researchers, the full-throttle zombie is a gold mine of disease information.

If a full-throttle zombie is part of a research study and begins Total Recovery, they'd get healthy and cause a skew in the research data. They'd put researchers in an awkward position.

The researchers would have to put a big asterisk in the middle of their data plot and say, "Hey, this is when TR skewed everything up." They don't want a skewed up data plot with a big asterisk. They want the full-throttle zombie to keep doing what they do best.

Second, doctors and surgery centers need the full-throttle zombie. They don't want the full-throttle zombie to start TR and get healthy. They need somebody to request expensive medicines and expensive surgical operations.

Third, researchers in the medical device and pharmaceutical industries need the full-throttle zombie. They don't want the full-throttle zombie to start TR and get healthy. They need someone to buy their artificial joints and their expensive pharmaceuticals.

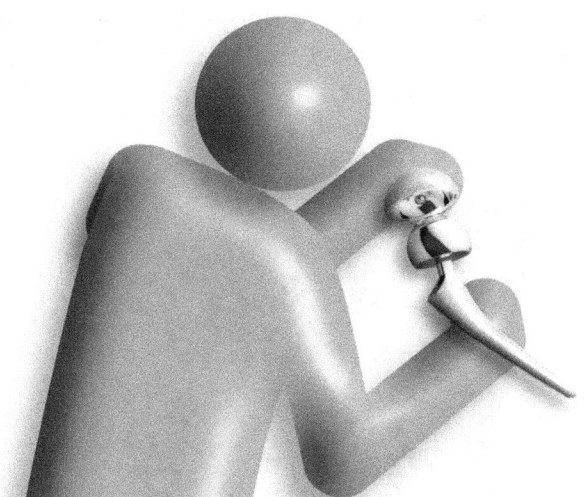

Someone to buy artificial joints.

Fourth, the sales reps in these industries need the full-throttle zombie. They don't want the full-throttle zombie to start TR and get healthy. They would miss their sales goals.

Every member of the entire healthcare industry wants the full-throttle zombie to keep doing what they do best.

FOR FULL-THROTTLE ZOMBIES ONLY

It should now be crystal-clear how TR defines the full-throttle zombie. It should also be clear whether you should or should NOT be reading this section. It is intended for full-throttle zombies <u>only</u>.

As a full-throttle zombie, you are granted full permission to read this book. However, before you begin a journey to TR, you must agree to the following terms of use.

First, you must agree to the following motivational techniques employed by this book: SATIRE,[**29**] IRONY,[**30**] and REVERSE PSYCHOLOGY.[**31**]

These motivational techniques can be deceptively sophisticated. Your failure to recognize these techniques may cause UNINTENDED personal insult and offense. You must understand the rationale for these techniques and not allow your feelings to get hurt. You have to see the big picture before you begin TR. You can't just think about yourself.

Second, you must get your doctor's permission. Every self-help book about health contains this warning. However, no other self-help book requires you to agree to satire, irony and reverse psychology. This book has different reasons for why you must get your doctor's permission.

Your doctor contributes to your prosperity, and, more importantly, you contribute to your doctor's prosperity. With TR, you will adjust YOUR LIFESTYLE, and you will get healthy. You will contribute less to your doctor's prosperity, so your doctor may need to adjust THEIR LIFESTYLE. To be considerate, you must get your doctor's permission.

Your doctor may rely on the prescriptions you fill at the pharmacy. Your doctor may receive kickbacks, provided by a pharmaceutical company for each of your filled prescriptions, to support their travel and vacation expenses.[**32**] You must get your doctor's permission, so they can budget their travel and vacation expenses.

Your doctor is your main point of contact with the massive health care food chain that feeds on your full-throttle zombie be-

---

29   Wikipedia. **Satire.** Accessed 2016. *en.wikipedia.org/wiki/Satire*

30   Wikipedia. **Irony.** Accessed 2016. *en.wikipedia.org/wiki/Irony*

31   Wikipedia. **Reverse psychology.** Accessed 2016. *en.wikipedia.org/wiki/Reverse_psychology*

32   Wikipedia. **Pharmaceutical fraud.** Accessed 2016. *en.wikipedia.org/wiki/Pharmaceutical_fraud*

haviors. When you become more healthy and stop filling your prescriptions, your doctor may get a call from their pharmaceutical sales reps asking why. Your doctor may need to explain to them that his patients are beginning TR. Your doctor may need to update the prescription writing goals that they've negotiated with their pharmaceutical sales reps. And, in turn, their sales reps may need to update the prescription sales goals that they've negotiated with their regional managers, and so on.

To be considerate to all the people in the health care system relying on your current lifestyle, you will need to get your doctor's permission before you begin a journey to TR. You have to see the big picture. You can't just think about yourself.

CHAPTER TWO REVIEW

Biological zombie. It's a creature in nature controlled by a pathogen. A biological zombie adopts behaviors that undermine its health while providing benefits to the pathogen.

Zombie behavior. It's a human behavior that undermines our long-term health or the health of the environment. This behavior is often encouraged by a third party and may even provide benefit to the third party.

Recovery behavior. It's a human behavior that preserves our long-term health and the health of the environment.

Zombie virus. It's a transmissible belief that promotes zombie behaviors. It's passed by advertisers, broadcast media, social media, and fellow infected people.

Normal zombies. They represent typical members of Western society. They understand the importance of health and the environment, yet they engage in zombie behaviors. They contribute to the looming non-communicable disease and climate change crises.

Recovering zombies. They represent followers of Total Recovery. They engage in mostly recovery behaviors and few zombie behaviors. They contribute little to the non-communicable disease and climate change crises.

Full-throttle zombies. They represent pleasure seekers and thrill seekers in Western society. They engage in few recovery behaviors and mostly zombie behaviors. They contribute disproportionately to the looming non-communicable disease and climate change crises.

Journey to recovery. This lifestyle intervention neutralizes zombie viruses, reduces zombie behaviors, and increases recovery behaviors. It utilizes various techniques to shield us from advertisers, broadcast media, social media, and infected people. Techniques include mindfulness, visualization, imagination, humor, irony, satire, and reverse psychology.

METABOLIC FITNESS

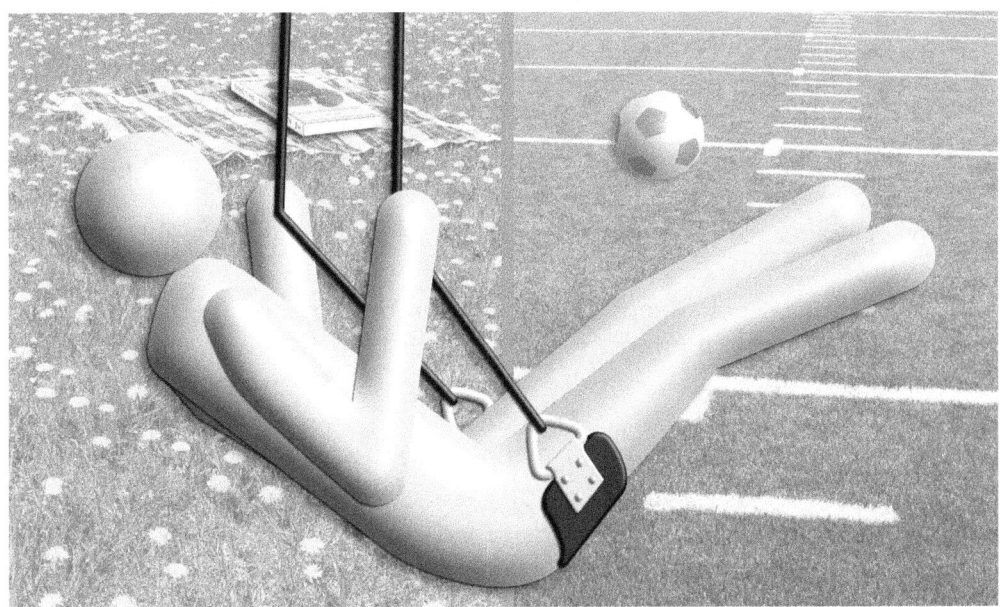

Metabolic activity swings between rest and exertion every day.

When most of us think about fitness, we think of physical fitness and we imagine a person jogging. Of the five fitnesses, physical fitness is mostly associated with metabolic fitness. We think of metabolic fitness first because it's most visible.

TR provides the metaphor of a dimmer switch of fitness to remind us that all five fitnesses are essential to total fitness. TR provides another metaphor called the *Swing of Activity* for each fitness. The Swing represents the complete range of daily activities pertinent to each form of fitness.

In this chapter, we discuss the following topics:

- *From metabolic fitness to frailty.*
- *What metabolic fitness looks like.*
- *What metabolic frailty looks like.*
- *The Swing of Metabolic Activity.*

- *Measuring metabolic fitness.*
- *The Dimmer Switch of Metabolic Fitness.*
- *Review.*

FROM METABOLIC FITNESS TO FRAILTY

Metabolism is the complete set of chemical reactions needed for the ecosystem of cells in our bodies. Metabolism includes the following processes: storing energy from food; burning energy from food; building up complex molecules for repair; breaking down complex molecules for removal; growing new cells to add to tissues; destroying damaged cells to remove from tissues; and regulating all these processes.[33]

Regulation happens to be the most important metabolic process. It's also the most vulnerable. It's effectiveness depends on how well we regulate our diet and our physical activity. When we fail to regulate our diet and physical activity, we cause our body's regulation of metabolism to fail. We cause metabolic disorders such as obesity, diabetes, cardiovascular disease, and cancer.

Our metabolic fitness tends to fade so gradually, we lose track of how much we've lost and how much worse it can get. We need to see the big picture to keep track of what's going on.

TR has developed the concept of metabolic fitness to help us see the big picture. Metabolic fitness is based on the VARIATION in metabolic ACTIVITY. It's represented in the *Metabolic Fitness And Activity Plot* below. If the concept and the plot work as designed, they should help us see where we are now and motivate us to try harder with diet and exercise.

The vertical axis on the plot represents metabolic activity. It varies from a low value when the body is at rest to a high value when the body is exercising.

The squiggly line on the plot can be imagined as the daily back and forth of the *Swing of Metabolic Activity*. It swings from a state of rest to a state of exertion. When we exercise every day, our swing carves a wide path. When we neglect daily exercise, our swing etches a tiny path.

---

33   Wikipedia. **Metabolism.** Accessed 2016. *en.wikipedia.org/wiki/Metabolism*

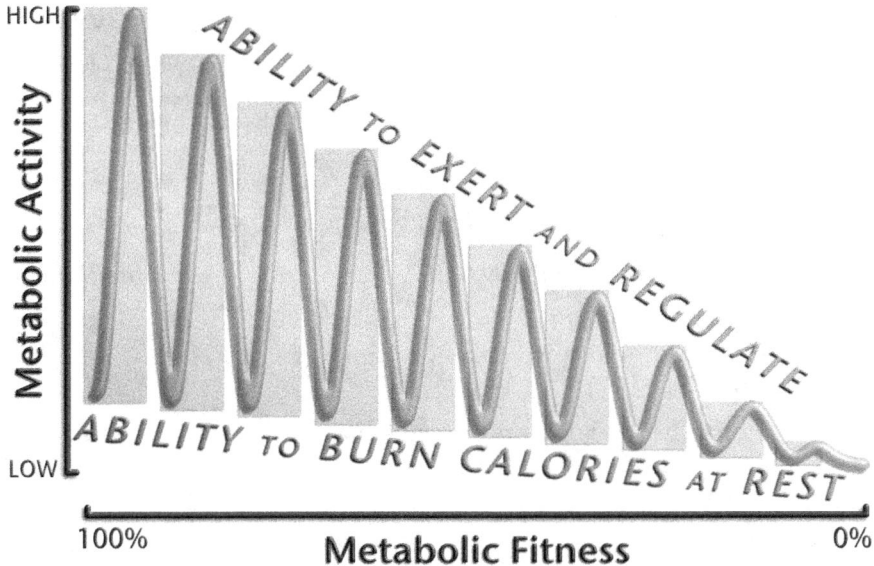

METABOLIC FITNESS AND ACTIVITY PLOT

Metabolic Fitness

The horizontal axis represents metabolic fitness. Fitness is highest when the daily back and forth swing of metabolic activity is widest. At 100% metabolic fitness, the body has the greatest ability for physical exertion, metabolic regulation, and burning calories at rest. The body has the most muscle tissue and the least fat tissue.

The vertical bars on the plot represent intervals of metabolic fitness. Each bar can be imagined as a snapshot of the *Dimmer Switch of Metabolic Fitness* that is slowly shutting off. We can push the dimmer higher with diet and exercise.

The top edge of the plot represents the body's fading ability for physical exertion and metabolic regulation as muscle is replaced by fat. The bottom edge of the plot represents the body's fading ability to burn calories at rest as muscle is replaced by fat.

WHAT METABOLIC FITNESS LOOKS LIKE

In the *Metabolic Fitness and Activity Plot* above, maximum metabolic fitness is depicted by the tallest bar on the far left, when the ability to exert and regulate metabolism is maximum, and the ability to burn calories at rest is maximum. Metabolic fitness represents resilience to the following sources of stress:

Exertion stress. It's the stress on our bodies when we engage in physical activity. Our heart, lungs, and muscles need to work together. Too much exertion stress can give us a heart attack. Here are examples of how resilience changes across different levels of metabolic fitness.

RESILIENCE TO EXERTION STRESS

%Fit	The Body Can	Health Risks
100%	Sprint at full speed, lift itself completely off the ground, and comfortably perform unusual activities.	None.
50%	Jog briefly, easily get down on the floor and back up, and comfortably perform ordinary activities.	Increased risk for metabolic disorder.
25%	Walk for short distances, slowly get down on the floor and back up, and cautiously perform ordinary activities.	Increased risk for metabolic disease and cancer.
1%	Barely sustain the effort to keep organs alive.	Death.

Macronutrient stress. It's the stress on our bodies when we over eat or under eat macronutrients. Most of us suffer from macronutrient excess. Refined carbohydrates and sugars elevate blood sugar.[34] Saturated fat from meat and dairy elevate blood cholesterol and triglyceride levels.[35] Protein from meat and dairy elevate blood calcium and increase risk of kidney stones.[36] Persistent macronutrient excess causes our organs to become frail. Here are examples of how resilience changes across different levels of metabolic fitness.

---

34 Wikipedia. **Insulin_resistance.** Accessed 2016. *en.wikipedia.org/wiki/Insulin_resistance*

35 Wikipedia. **Combined_hyperlipidemia.** Accessed 2016. *en.wikipedia.org/wiki/Combined_hyperlipidemia*

36 Wikipedia. **Kidney_stone.** Accessed 2016. *en.wikipedia.org/wiki/Kidney_stone*

RESILIENCE TO MACRONUTRIENT STRESS

%Fit	Refined Carbs or Sugar	Fat From Meat or Dairy	Protein From Meat Or Dairy
100%	Regulated blood glucose.	Regulated blood fats.	Regulated protein metabolites.
25%	Elevated blood glucose and insulin resistance.	Elevated blood fats, including LDL and triglycerides.	Elevated protein metabolites and kidney stones.

DNA damage stress. It's the stress on each cell in our bodies. Every cell suffers DNA damage throughout the day that needs to be repaired. Remarkably, our cells sustain up to one million events of DNA damage every single day.[37] DNA damage stress is caused by macronutrients, carcinogens, radiation, and insufficient repair, as follows.

Macronutrients. DNA damage is caused by reactive metabolites formed during the incomplete burning of carbohydrates and fats. These metabolites form when we eat too much and move too little. [38] It's like when an engine or a campfire is given too much fuel and not enough oxygen, causing the formation of noxious pollution.

Carcinogens. DNA damage is caused by carcinogens formed in grilled food[39] and by carcinogens released by pathogenic bacteria which are fostered in the gut by processed foods.[40]

Radiation. DNA damage is caused by UV radiation from sun exposure.[41]

Insufficient repair. Every cell needs time to repair DNA damage. Insufficient repair can occur when the rate of damage increases

37   Wikipedia. **DNA repair.** Accessed 2016. *en.wikipedia.org/wiki/DNA_repair*

38   Wikipedia. **Oxidative stress.** Accessed 2016. *en.wikipedia.org/wiki/Oxidative_stress*

39   Wikipedia. **Heterocyclic amine formation in meat.** Accessed 2016. *en.wikipedia.org/wiki/Heterocyclic_amine_formation_in_meat*

40   Wikipedia. **Pathogenic Escherichia coli.** Accessed 2016. *en.wikipedia.org/wiki/Pathogenic_Escherichia_coli*

41   Wikipedia. **Direct DNA damage.** Accessed 2016. *en.wikipedia.org/wiki/Direct_DNA_damage*

from multiple sources simultaneously. It can occur when the rate of repair decreases — for instance, by missing nightly DNA repair.

Here is a summary of DNA damage stresses that lead to decreased metabolic fitness.

SOURCES OF DNA DAMAGE STRESS

Macronutrients	Refined carbs and fats.
Carcinogens	Grilled food and pathogenic gut bacteria fostered by processed foods.
Radiation	Sun exposure.
Insufficient repair	Cumulative stresses and insufficient nightly repair.

WHAT METABOLIC FRAILTY LOOKS LIKE

In the *Metabolic Fitness and Activity Plot* above, maximum metabolic frailty is depicted by the shortest bar on the far right. At this point, the body loses the ability for physical exertion beyond the minimum needed to rest, maintain organ function, and repair DNA.

Metabolic frailty increases the risk of the following conditions:

Cancer. One-half of cancer deaths are attributed to diet, physical inactivity, and obesity.[42] Upwards of 70% to 90% of cancers are attributed to avoidable factors, such as lifestyle and environment, and not genetic factors.[43]

Dementia. The second most common form of dementia is attributed to a declining supply of blood to the brain and is known as vascular dementia.[44]

Frailty. The progressive loss of weight, muscle, bone, and energy is attributed to the declining ability for physical exertion and metabolic regulation.[45]

---

42   Song M, Giovannucci E. **Preventable Incidence and Mortality of Carcinoma Associated With Lifestyle Factors Among White Adults in the United States.** JAMA Oncol. 2016 May 19. *pubmed.gov/27196525*

43   Wu S, Hannun Y. **The importance of extrinsic factors in the development of cancers.** Mol Cell Oncol. 2016 Feb 24;3(3):e1143079. *pubmed.gov/27314092*

44   Wikipedia. **Vascular dementia.** Accessed 2016. *en.wikipedia.org/wiki/Vascular_dementia*

45   Wikipedia. **Frailty syndrome.** Accessed 2016. *en.wikipedia.org/wiki/*

Wasting. The dramatic loss of weight, muscle, energy, and appetite is attributed to cancer and declining organ function. The clinical term is cachexia.[**46**]

Heart stops. Cardiac arrest is attributed to a dramatic loss in the capacity for any physical exertion and metabolic regulation.[**47**]

Heart and lungs stop. Clinical death is attributed to a dramatic loss in the capacity for any physical exertion and metabolic regulation.[**48**]

Metabolic frailty is the straw that breaks the camel's back and causes death by natural causes. None of the other forms of frailty can cause immediate death all by themselves. They each induce metabolic frailty and indirectly cause death by natural causes. Immune frailty is the one exception because it causes metabolic frailty so quickly. In the case of septic shock, its effects are practically instantaneous.

THE SWING OF METABOLIC ACTIVITY

The *Swing of Metabolic Activity* is a visual metaphor to remind us to put in effort every single day.

The Metabolic Fitness And Activity Plot uses a squiggly line to represent the daily arc of the Swing of Metabolic Activity. As we proceed through calendar years, our swing loses momentum, and its daily arc shortens.

When we notice our fading ability for exertion and other symptoms of metabolic disorder, we visit our doctor. We ask him to give us a push on our swing. Well, frankly, we pay him to give us a push. He obliges, but he may not give us the right kind of push.

Sometimes, he pushes our swing at the wrong part of its

Frailty_syndrome

46   Wikipedia. **Cachexia.** Accessed 2016. *en.wikipedia.org/wiki/Cachexia*

47   Wikipedia. **Cardiac arrest.** Accessed 2016. *en.wikipedia.org/wiki/Cardiac_arrest*

48   Wikipedia. **Clinical death.** Accessed 2016. *en.wikipedia.org/wiki/Clinical_death*

arc, and he mistakenly slows us down. We might shrug it off, or we might complain about him to our friends. We probably start shopping for a different doctor.

What we really need to do is pump our swing ourselves. We must commit ourselves to exercising and eating healthy foods every day.

We have to pump our swing with the right force and the right rhythm. When we pump incorrectly, we end up with a sore tendon or a sore tummy. We must push ourselves to exercise hard, but not push our bodies too far too fast. We must transition to new foods, but not push our tummies too far too fast.

Pumping our swing takes finesse, timing, and perseverance.

MEASURING METABOLIC FITNESS

We tend to think we can assess the metabolic fitness of a person based on folds of fat or mounds of muscle. But these things are motionless features, and metabolic fitness represents a dynamic property of the body. We can only INFER metabolic fitness from motionless features.

Fitness must be measured by how well the body accommodates stress — it's resilience to stress. Few health assessments measure the body's resilience to stress. Typical health measurements such as body weight, percent body fat, heart rate, blood pressure, and blood sugar are taken when the body is at rest.

Researchers measure metabolic activity directly by measuring RESPIRATION. Respiration is how much oxygen we breathe in and how much carbon dioxide we breathe out. The technique is called respirometry.[49]

Respirometry is a lot like testing the tailpipe emissions on a car. A technician asks us to breathe in and out through a tube connected to a sensor that measures our oxygen consumption and our carbon dioxide emission.

Resting metabolic rate. A respiratory technician can use our

49　Wikipedia. **Respirometry.** Accessed 2016. *en.wikipedia.org/wiki/ Respirometry* oxygen consumption and carbon dioxide emission to estimate our ability to burn calories at rest. Respiratory technicians refer to this quantity as the resting metabolic rate.[50] Resting metabolic rate is the same as our ability to burn calories at rest. It corresponds to the bottom edge of each vertical bar on the *Metabolic Fitness and Activity Plot*.

Maximum metabolic rate. A respiratory technician can use our oxygen consumption and carbon dioxide emission while we are jogging on a treadmill to estimate our ability for physical exertion. Respiratory technicians denote the volume of oxygen consumed at maximum exertion as VO_{2max}.[51] VO_{2max} is the same as our ability for physical exertion. It corresponds to the top edge of each vertical bar on the *Metabolic Fitness and Activity Plot*.

VO2max represents our maximum lung capacity, blood flow, heart function, and muscle capacity. It represents the resilience of the entire cardiorespiratory and musculoskeletal systems to exertion stress. The only thing that helps us improve our VO_{2max} is daily exercise. It's really hard to fake it out. The measurement of VO_{2max} is a real-world stress test for metabolic fitness.

Here's a snapshot of the research studies that confirm the importance of metabolic fitness.

Metabolic fitness of men. University of Colorado Boulder researchers examine how VO_{2max} declines with calendar age and lack of exercise in men. The researchers pool the data from 242 prior studies and create a dataset of around 14,000 men who range in calendar age from 20 to 80 years old. The researchers group the men into three groups: men who exercise almost daily, men who exercise weekly, and men who exercise rarely.[52]

When the researchers compare the men within the SAME exercise group, the researchers observe that VO2max DECLINES with calendar age while body fat INCREASES with calendar age. When

50   Wikipedia. **Resting metabolic rate.** Accessed 2016. *en.wikipedia.org/ wiki/Resting_metabolic_rate*

51   Wikipedia. **VO2 max.** Accessed 2016. *en.wikipedia.org/wiki/VO2_ max*

52   Wilson TM, Tanaka H. **Meta-analysis of the age-associated decline in maximal aerobic capacity in men: relation to training status.** Am J Physiol Heart Circ Physiol. 2000 Mar;278(3):H829-34. *pubmed.gov/ 10710351*

the researchers compare the men in DIFFERENT exercise groups, they observe that the DAILY exercising men in their 60s have greater VO2max values and less body fat than the RARELY exercising men in their 20s.

Metabolic fitness of women. University of Colorado Boulder researchers also examine how VO_{2max} declines with calendar age and lack of exercise in women. The researchers pool the data from 109 prior studies and create a dataset of around 5,000 women who range in calendar age from 20 to 80 years old. The researchers group the women into three groups: women who exercise almost daily, women who exercise weekly, and women who exercise rarely.[53]

When the researchers compare the women within the SAME exercise group, the researchers observe that VO2max DECLINES with calendar age. When the researchers compare the women in DIFFERENT exercise groups, they observe that the DAILY exercising women in their 50s have greater VO2max values than the RARELY exercising women in their 20s.

THE DIMMER SWITCH OF METABOLIC FITNESS

The *Dimmer Switch of Metabolic Fitness* is a visual metaphor to remind us what's at stake.

In metabolic youth, our Dimmer Switch of Metabolic Fitness starts at the highest setting. As we proceed through calendar years, our dimmer switch slides downward.

If we pump our Swing of Metabolic Activity, we can kick our dimmer switch higher. But we have to kick it constantly. In between kicks, it resumes its slow slide downward.

Without daily exercise, a person's ability for physical exertion will always shrink. A person may be 100% DISEASE-FREE their ENTIRE life, yet their ability for

---

53   Fitzgerald MD, Tanaka H, Tran ZV, Seals DR. **Age-related declines in maximal aerobic capacity in regularly exercising vs. sedentary women: a meta-analysis.** J Appl Physiol (1985). 1997 Jul;83(1):160-5. *pubmed.gov/9216959*

physical exertion will fade until it equals their ability to burn calories at rest.

When a person cannot muster the exertion to do anything more than rest, they really can't do anything for themselves. Their Dimmer Switch of Metabolic Fitness is at the point where the light is flickering.

The loss of metabolic fitness is the ultimate arbiter of biological age and death by natural causes.

If your buttons are getting pushed in all the right places by the swing and the dimmer switch metaphors, then you may begin questioning all the exercise-o-phobic defenses you've built to protect yourself. You may wonder if these defenses are weighing down your swing and your dimmer switch. You may wish to begin pumping your swing and kicking your dimmer switch higher.

You'll want to start thinking about exercise and how to measure your VO_{2max}. If you prefer machines and technology, you can measure your VO_{2max} in a sports medicine clinic or a respirometry lab. But you don't need to. You can use questionnaires on the internet to get a reasonable estimate.

TR recommends this particular online questionnaire developed by Norwegian researchers.[54] This questionnaire is validated by published research studies. It gathers information about your exercise routine, lifestyle, and body shape to estimate VO_{2max}. It also reports the age of people who typically have that same value, which is something like an estimate of your biological age. The Norwegian researchers show their VO_{2max} estimate can predict cardiovascular as well as all-cause mortality.[55]

The questionnaire about exercise and lifestyle will help you prioritize how to increase your VO_{2max}, how to pump your swing higher, and how to kick your dimmer switch higher.

Happy swinging.

54   World Fitness Level website. **How fit are you, really?** Accessed 2016. *worldfitnesslevel.org*

55   Nes BM, Vatten LJ, Nauman J, Janszky I, Wisløff U. **A simple nonexercise model of cardiorespiratory fitness predicts long-term mortality.** Med Sci Sports Exerc. 2014 Jun;46(6):1159-65. *pubmed.gov/24576863*

CHAPTER THREE REVIEW

Metabolism. Metabolism is the complete set of chemical reactions needed for biological life. Metabolism includes burning energy from food, storing energy from food, building up complex molecules for repair, breaking down complex molecules for removal, and most importantly, regulating all these reactions. The effectiveness of metabolic regulation depends on how well we regulate our diet and our physical activity.

Resting metabolic rate. It's the rate at which our bodies burn calories while we're resting. It's measured by the volume of oxygen we consume at rest. It increases when we build muscle. It decreases when we lose muscle or when our muscle tissue becomes invaded by fat cells.

VO2max. It's the maximum volume of oxygen we consume at full exertion. It represents the maximum rate at which our bodies can burn calories. It's also our maximum rate of metabolism. It increases with exercise training. It decreases with lack of exercise. When it equals our resting metabolic rate, our bodies can no longer sustain the effort to live.

ZOMBIE VIRUSES

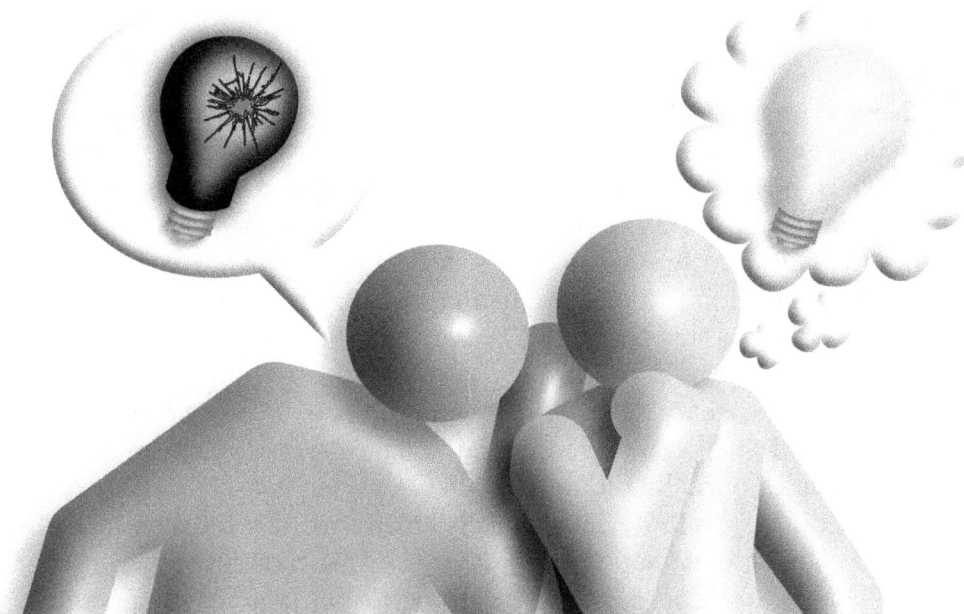

Advertisers whisper bad ideas that sound to us like good ideas.

Our minds are often polluted with bad ideas. People whisper bad ideas to us, and we mistakenly think they're good ideas. Advertisers constantly whisper bad ideas to us. The entire advertising industry is based on taking bad ideas — that they know are bad ideas — and making us think they're good ideas.

These bad ideas can be imagined as zombie viruses that infect our minds and that short-circuit our mindfulness and our decision making. They are transmitted from person to person like pathogens. They cause us to engage in zombie behaviors that undermine our long-term health and the health of the environment.

In this chapter, we examine the following topics:
- *The therapeutic happiness virus.*
- *Therapeutic happiness shortens lifespan.*
- *Conscientiousness extends lifespan.*

- *The annoying conscientiousness virus.*
- *The anything but exercise virus.*
- *The high protein virus.*
- *The quick-fix virus.*
- *Review.*

THE **THERAPEUTIC HAPPINESS VIRUS**

Everyone has a notion that happiness is so therapeutic it can justify unhealthy behaviors. This notion is a zombie virus. It's lodged deep in our minds. It's also lodged deep in our zombie culture and in our zombie health care system. It's endemic to Western society.

Because we think "happiness is therapeutic," we freely adopt zombie behaviors in pursuit of happiness. We encourage our friends to join us in zombie behaviors, or we chide them for being virtuous goody two-shoes.

We often hear that happiness is so therapeutic, it helps us fight cancer and attain a longer lifespan. When psychologists study the personalities of really old people, they routinely tell us how important happiness is.[**56**] Unfortunately, there are a few flaws in the logic of therapeutic happiness promoted by psychologists.

Happy and sad movies. According to the logic of therapeutic happiness, happy and sad movies should affect our health. Watching happy movies should increase our happiness, increase our healthiness, and increase our lifespans. Conversely, watching sad movies should decrease our happiness, decrease our healthiness, and decrease our lifespans. If these effects were real, we would need health warnings on all movies, television shows, and books with sad endings to let us make informed decisions. Of course, this scenario is completely preposterous. Therapeutic happiness is illogical.

Wrong study subjects. Psychologists promoting therapeutic happiness are generally studying the wrong people. When they study really old people, they may be observing an increase in happiness as an EFFECT that arises from differences in survivorship.[**57**]

---

56   Frey BS. **Psychology. Happy people live longer.** Science. 2011 Feb 4;331(6017):542-3. *pubmed.gov/21292959*

57   Segerstrom SC, Combs HL, Winning A, Boehm JK, Kubzansky LD. **The**

What they need to do, instead, is measure the happiness of young people and test whether differences in happiness CAUSE differences in survival.

Healthiness and happiness. UK researchers run the right experiment — with the right group of people — to test whether happiness leads to health and longevity.[58] They study almost a million women for over 10 years. At the beginning of the study, they ask the women, who are around 59 years old, to report their state of healthiness and their state of happiness. They notice that women who report low healthiness tend to report low happiness, and women who report high healthiness tend to report high happiness.

During the 10 years of the study, the UK researchers observe that deaths can be linked back to the initial self-reported HEALTHINESS, pre-existing medical conditions, and sociodemographic factors. The researchers see no evidence that self-reported HAPPINESS helps to further explain deaths. The researchers provide evidence that pursuing happiness does not bring health. It's the other way around. PURSUING HEALTH BRINGS HAPPINESS. If we want to be happy, we have to be healthy first.

We have the cause-and-effect backwards. Our own health care community — especially our psychologists — tell us that happiness causes healthiness. Everybody believes happiness will nurture our health. The therapeutic happiness virus is endemic to our zombie society. It's so virulent, we can remove it one day, and it simply re-infects us the next day. This virus requires our constant vigilance.

THERAPEUTIC HAPPINESS SHORTENS LIFESPAN

Imagine we could test the idea of therapeutic happiness with a study that runs even longer than 10 years? Perhaps one that lasts a whole lifetime?

happy survivor? Effects of differential mortality on life satisfaction in older age. Psychol Aging. 2016 Jun;31(4):340-5. *pubmed.gov/27294716*

58   Liu B, Floud S, Pirie K, Green J, Peto R, Beral V; Million Women Study Collaborators. **Does happiness itself directly affect mortality? The prospective UK Million Women Study.** Lancet. 2015 Dec 9. pii: S0140-6736(15)01087-9. *pubmed.gov/26684609*

Imagine we could study 10 year olds and group them according to whether they have a happy demeanor or an unhappy demeanor. Imagine we could follow the happy children their entire lives to see whether they survive longer. Of course, we would all assume they'd live longer. We'd be willing to bet money on it. But we'd all be wrong.

Terman study. Back in 1922, Lewis Terman at Stanford University began such a study testing the happiness and the future lifespan of 10 year olds. The Terman Life Cycle Study enrolled over 1,000 children, profiled their IQs, profiled their personalities, and then monitored them their entire lives.[**59**]

Terman study at 70 years. Seventy years into the study, researchers examine the personality and survival data.[**60**] They notice that happy demeanor provides no survival advantage. Boys with a happy demeanor tend to die sooner. Boys with a serious demeanor tend to live longer.

It's the complete opposite of what we all expect. But when we think about it — hard enough — it makes perfect sense. Being care-*FREE* fosters a care*LESS* lifestyle. Being SERIOUS fosters a SENSIBLE lifestyle.

Preventative seriousness always makes more sense, and yet the therapeutic happiness virus keeps infecting our minds. It feels so good in there. It lets us rationalize so many zombie behaviors in the name of health. We convince ourselves we're smarter than the virtuous goody two-shoes. Therapeutic happiness is the perfect zombie virus.

We've known the therapeutic happiness virus for so long, it's become a close friend. We'll defend it to the death — no matter how many times it lets us down. It's what friends do for each other.

CONSCIENTIOUSNESS EXTENDS LIFESPAN

The Terman Life Cycle Study is generating personality and survival

59   Wikipedia. **Lewis Terman.** Accessed 2016. *en.wikipedia.org/wiki/Lewis_Terman*

60   Schwartz JE, Friedman HS, Tucker JS, Tomlinson-Keasey C, Wingard DL, Criqui MH. **Sociodemographic and psychosocial factors in childhood as predictors of adult mortality.** Am J Public Health. 1995 Sep; 85(9):1237-45. *pubmed.gov/7661231*

data that refutes the therapeutic happiness virus. The study also reveals the real secret to survival: the conscientious personality trait.

Terman study at 80 years. Eighty years into the Terman Study, researchers at University of California Riverside report that childhood conscientiousness predicts lifetime survival.[61] They also report adulthood conscientiousness predicts survival.

Confirmatory study. In a separate study of conscientious boys, the researchers confirm a nearly 20% boost in lifetime survival.[62]

Decreases mortality. UK researchers examine how lack of conscientiousness influences early death.[63] In a group of nearly 7,000 adults, they observe a 10% decrease in mortality for each standard deviation increase in conscientiousness.

Increases longevity. Finnish researchers examine how personality influences longevity.[64] They perform a meta-analysis of seven studies totaling 76,000 adults. Of all the personality traits measured, only conscientiousness is significant. More conscientiousness produces a 40% higher longevity.

Reduces high-risk behaviors. Psychiatric researchers examine how conscientiousness reduces high-risk health behaviors and mortality.[65] They analyze 14-year mortality data on over 6,000 adults.

61 Martin LR, Friedman HS, Schwartz JE. **Personality and mortality risk across the life span: the importance of conscientiousness as a biopsychosocial attribute.** Health Psychol. 2007 Jul;26(4):428-36. *pubmed.gov/17605562*

62 Kern ML, Friedman HS, Martin LR, Reynolds CA, Luong G. **Conscientiousness, career success, and longevity: a lifespan analysis.** Ann Behav Med. 2009 Apr;37(2):154-63. *pubmed.gov/19455378*

63 Hagger-Johnson G, Sabia S, Nabi H, Brunner E, Kivimaki M, Shipley M, Singh-Manoux A. **Low conscientiousness and risk of all-cause, cardiovascular and cancer mortality over 17 years: Whitehall II cohort study.** J Psychosom Res. 2012 Aug;73(2):98-103. *pubmed.gov/22789411*

64 Jokela M, Batty GD, Nyberg ST, Virtanen M, Nabi H, Singh-Manoux A, Kivimäki M. **Personality and all-cause mortality: individual-participant meta-analysis of 3,947 deaths in 76,150 adults.** Am J Epidemiol. 2013 Sep 1;178(5):667-75. *pubmed.gov/23911610*

65 Turiano NA, Chapman BP, Gruenewald TL, Mroczek DK. **Personality and the leading behavioral contributors of mortality.** Health Psychol. 2015 Jan;34(1):51-60. *pubmed.gov/24364374*

They observe more conscientiousness reduces heavy drinking, smoking, and waist circumference, leading to a 13% reduction in death.

Conscientiousness gives a powerful boost to longevity because it fosters discipline, impulse control, and responsibility to others. It is a personality trait that we associate with eating sensible foods, eating sensible portions, eating at regular meal times, brushing and flossing teeth, going to bed and getting up on time, planning ahead, managing stress, and exercising regularly.[66] It's a personality trait that is built for the long haul, and not the short escapade.

Conscientiousness is cultivated by Total Recovery. And because conscientiousness is part of our personality, the journey to recovery requires changing part of our personality to increase our conscientiousness.

It may sound strange for us to think about changing our personalities. Personality change may sound strange and improbable at first. But we just have to ask ourselves: How do we assess other peoples' personalities? By their behaviors.

If a person has wild and crazy behaviors, we think they're a party animal. And if that person begins to take their health seriously and begins adopting healthy behaviors, we'll think they're no longer a party animal. We'll think they've matured and grown up. In other words, we'll think their personality has changed.

TR creates the concepts of zombie viruses and zombie behaviors to help put some distance between the party animal we once aspired to be and the mature and sensible person we WANT to be. It doesn't really matter what kind of personality we think we have right now. It only matters whether we want to reduce our zombie behaviors and adopt recovery behaviors. When we're ready to start our journey to recovery, TR will show us the path — behaviors, personality, and everything else.

THE ANNOYING CONSCIENTIOUSNESS VIRUS

We often don't like to think about conscientiousness because we're infected with the annoying conscientiousness virus. This zombie virus causes us to believe that people with conscientiousness per-

---

66   Wikipedia. **Conscientiousness.** Accessed 2016. *en.wikipedia.org/ wiki/Conscientiousness*

sonalities are annoying. We believe that when these people over-think their health, they stop having fun, they start getting less healthy, and they really annoy us in the process.

Conscientiousness is so annoying that we'll refer to it as the C word whenever possible. We'll refer to the zombie virus itself as the ANNOYING C WORD virus.

Health perfectionists. We associate the C word with health perfectionists. The annoying C word virus gives us permission to hassle health perfectionists. We call them goody two-shoes, nitpick-ers, fussbudgets, dorks, wussies, and pussies. We ridicule them be-cause they take the fun out of the bad things we like to do. We just want to have a party, but the health perfectionists are a buzz-kill.

We want health perfectionists to loosen up and live a little. This zombie virus makes us believe it's MORE healthy to do UN-HEALTHY things every so often. We think we're doing health per-fectionists a favor by hassling them.

Or, we just want them to go away. Perhaps, we may even want them to fail. We'd love to see a health perfectionist get sick. Then we can say to ourselves, "It look's like being so perfect isn't so good after all." The last thing we'll admit to ourselves is that the health perfectionists will be the ones at the high school reunion who keep looking healthy, young, and attractive.

Objects of ridicule. Our society is moving from an information society to an entertainment society. Hollywood movies are what we live and breathe. Hollywood movies will never celebrate the C word. They're about finding short-cuts, taking risks, flirting with be-ing bad, and being the life of the party.

If a Hollywood movie ever has a character representing the C word, they're always an object of ridicule. The C word character al-ways gets in the way of the main character. We root for the main character to outsmart the C word character. It cracks us up when a C word character gets put back in their place.

Consider our admiration of Benjamin Franklin who is attributed with this proverb about the C word:

"Early to bed and early to rise, makes a man healthy, wealthy and wise."[67]

---

67   Wikipedia. **Waking up early.** Accessed 2016. *en.wikipedia.org/wiki/ Waking_up_early*

We admire Benjamin Franklin for many reasons, but we don't admire him for this proverb. We admire him DESPITE this proverb. We wish he'd never said it. We try to ignore his proverb about the C word.

THE ANYTHING BUT EXERCISE VIRUS

This zombie virus makes us dwell on the negative aspects of exercise such as how it makes our bodies sweat, stink, and ache. This virus makes us fantasize about medications and surgeries to improve our health or our body shape.

When our body's metabolic regulation begins to fail, we expect our doctors to prescribe medications to bring down our blood pressure, our blood sugar, and our cholesterol. We expect our doctors to prescribe ANYTHING but exercise.

We know fat is bad. We consider surgeries to get rid of fat. We consider LIPO to suck fat right out of our bodies.[68] We consider putting a LAP-BAND around our stomachs.[69] We consider having our stomachs STAPLED.[70] We even consider putting a TOILET PUMP right inside our stomachs.[71] We are willing to try ANYTHING but exercise.

We know muscle is good. We fantasize surgeons will develop a procedure to graft new muscle. We fantasize researchers will develop a medication to grow new muscle. We think about ANYTHING but exercise.

Doctors are infected with this zombie virus too. They assess our health by measuring our weight, our blood pressure, and our heart rate. Doctors never assess our health by asking us to do a push-up, a pull-up, a plank, or a sit-up. Doctors never measure these things. They measure ANYTHING but exercise.

68   Wikipedia. **Liposuction.** Accessed 2016. *en.wikipedia.org/wiki/Liposuction*

69   Wikipedia. **Adjustable_gastric_band.** Accessed 2016. *en.wikipedia.org/wiki/Adjustable_gastric_band*

70   Wikipedia. **Vertical_banded_gastroplasty_surgery.** Accessed 2016. *en.wikipedia.org/wiki/Vertical_banded_gastroplasty_surgery*

71   Wikipedia. **Aspiration_therapy.** Accessed 2016. *en.wikipedia.org/wiki/Aspiration_therapy*

Doctors can't charge high fees for telling us to exercise. And we don't like paying large fees to doctors for telling us to exercise. And so, our doctors measure the easy stuff, they prescribe the expensive stuff, and we all go on with our day thinking about ANYTHING but exercise.

THE **HIGH PROTEIN VIRUS**

This virus makes us think protein is so important for health, we go out of our way to choose foods and snacks that are high in protein. It infects us when we're children because adults worry about our growth. It continues infecting us when we're adults even though we're done growing. It continues infecting us despite our fears of cancer and tumor growth.

Unfortunately, the Western diet is already supplying too much dietary protein and is contributing to metabolic frailty. Excess protein intake is associated with bone and calcium disorder, kidney stones and kidney disorder, cancer, liver disorder, and coronary artery disease.[72]

UCLA researchers observe that consumption of meat and dairy increases the risk of diabetes and cancer. They group 3,000 adults aged 50 to 65 according to low, medium, and high animal protein consumption. Over the course of 18 years, the high animal protein group has a 300% increase in cancer and diabetes mortality. The researchers observe that the boost in cancer mortality is like smoking cigarettes.[73]

The high protein virus makes us think high protein foods help us build muscle and bone, rather than kidney stones and cancer. It makes us want to consume meat, dairy, protein bars, and protein drinks. It makes us think animal-based foods are superior and plant-

---

72   Delimaris I. **Adverse Effects Associated with Protein Intake above the Recommended Dietary Allowance for Adults.** ISRN Nutr. 2013 Jul 18;2013:126929. *pubmed.gov/24967251*

73   Levine ME, Suarez JA, Brandhorst S, Balasubramanian P, Cheng CW, Madia F, Fontana L, Mirisola MG, Guevara-Aguirre J, Wan J, Passarino G, Kennedy BK, Wei M, Cohen P, Crimmins EM, Longo VD. **Low protein intake is associated with a major reduction in IGF-1, cancer, and overall mortality in the 65 and younger but not older population.** Cell Metab. 2014 Mar 4;19(3):407-17. *pubmed.gov/24606898*

based foods are deficient. It makes us think vegetarians and especially vegans are whacko.

The high protein virus makes us support new industries that supply high protein products. Greek-style yogurt has exploded in popularity based on its high protein content. Protein bars, protein shakes, and bodybuilding supplements are increasingly popular.

To combat this virus, we must weaken our association of high protein product with bone and muscle growth, and we must reinforce our association of high protein products with kidney stones, colorectal polyps,[74] and colorectal cancer growth.[75] To help us in this effort, TR provides a *High Protein Anti-Virus Translator* below. It helps us translate commonly marketed phrases with less attractive — but more accurate — phrases.

HIGH PROTEIN ANTI-VIRUS TRANSLATOR

"Stronger bones"	$\longrightarrow$	*"Bigger stones"*
"Muscle growth"	$\longrightarrow$	*"Cancer growth"*
"Protein bars"	$\longrightarrow$	*"Polyp bars"*
"Protein shakes"	$\longrightarrow$	*"Polyp shakes"*

One company takes the high protein virus to a comical extreme by selling a protein drink whose brandname combines the word MUSCLE and the word MILK. We should refer to their drink as "Malignant Milk." Coincidentally, consumer advocates report that "Malignant Milk" is actually packed with cancer-promoting heavy metals such as lead, arsenic, and cadmium, which the company fails to properly showcase on its label.[76] The high protein combined with the heavy metals mean that "Malignant Milk" might be the best "polyp shake" on the market for faster "cancer growth."

---

74   Wikipedia. **Colorectal polyp.** Accessed 2016. *en.wikipedia.org/wiki/Colorectal_polyp*

75   Wikipedia. **Colorectal cancer.** Accessed 2016. *en.wikipedia.org/wiki/Colorectal_cancer*

76   Wikipedia. **CytoSport.** Accessed 2016.   *en.wikipedia.org/wiki/CytoSport*

This virus makes us think that someday soon a high-tech medical breakthrough will erase our aging like a bogus Fountain of Youth. [77] This virus is spread by news reports about how high-tech medicine is getting closer to cures for the big diseases and for our aging.

High-tech medicine keeps assuring us that a quick-fix is around 10 years away. For some reason, news reporters never go back and research what was promised 10 years ago and hold high-tech medicine accountable for its unrealistic promises.

Nevertheless, the assurances from high-tech medicine help create the quick-fix virus which infects our minds and lulls us into complacency with our health. We wait like zombies for someone to fix what we've done to our bodies.

We need to question the quick-fix virus for the following reasons:

Aging is NOT a disease. Everyone hopes for a medication to quick-fix our aging. Yet medications always have SIDE EFFECTS. When we have a REAL disease, we are willing to tolerate the side effects of medications and surgeries. But if we are healthy and simply getting older, we will have much less tolerance for side effects.

Aging is a side effect. Aging is itself a side effect of the body's loss of fitness and gain of frailty. One of the most troubling effect of aging is how the body becomes more vulnerable to the side effects of medications as it becomes more frail.

Trading side effects. Any potential medication for aging won't cure our underlying frailty. It will just be treating a side effect of our frailty. And while it treats one side effect, it will cause other unknown side effects. We will simply be trading a side effect of frailty for other unknown side effects.

Mediocre medications. A medication for aging will likely be mediocre because its unknown side-effects may be as bad as aging itself. Many purportedly safe over-the-counter medications we take every day have recently been discovered to have age-accelerating side effects. We will discuss the under-reported side-effects of pain relievers and acid reflux medications in *Book Two: Biological Hap-*

---

77   Wikipedia. **Fountain of Youth.** Accessed 2016. *en.wikipedia.org/wiki/Fountain_of_Youth*

piness.

Dangerous medications. Johns Hopkins University researchers estimate that medical errors are the third leading cause of death in the US after heart disease and cancer.[78] They estimate that surgical errors and medication errors cause 250,000 deaths per year in the US. No government agency tracks deaths caused by medical mistakes, so nobody knows the actual number.

The quick-fix virus causes us to surrender responsibility for our health. We stop maintaining our fitness. We surrender to frailty. We assume all the smart people out there are going to find the quick fix for aging. We don't realize all those smart people are infected with the same quick-fix virus that infects us.

We have to fight the quick-fix virus just like we have to fight all the other zombie viruses that seduce us with fantasy and lull us into complacency.

---

78   Makary MA, Daniel M. **Medical error-the third leading cause of death in the US.** BMJ. 2016 May 3;353:i2139. *pubmed.gov/ 27143499*

CHAPTER FOUR REVIEW

Zombie virus. It's a bad idea someone tells us that we, in turn, think is a good idea. It's created by marketers and delivered to us by pervasive advertising. It encourages us to use a product and to adopt an unhealthy lifestyle. It contributes to the epidemic of non-communicable disease and premature death. It's so powerful that all health advice will fail unless the zombie virus is specifically identified and neutralized.

Therapeutic happiness virus. This zombie virus makes us believe that happiness by ITSELF boosts our mental health and somehow trickles down and improves our physical health. It makes us think that UNHEALTHY behaviors will generate sufficient HAPPINESS to actually become THERAPEUTIC.

This virus makes us encourage other people to share zombie behaviors with us. When we share a zombie behavior, we think the shared experience generates GREATER HAPPINESS and becomes MORE THERAPEUTIC.

This virus weakens our judgment. It makes us vulnerable to the unhealthy influence of family, friends, celebrities, and advertisers. This virus is endemic to Western society.

This virus is dangerous because it confuses the effect with the cause. Researchers show that healthiness causes happiness, not the other way around. Researchers also show that pursuing happiness actually shortens lifespan. On the other hand, they show that seriousness — not happiness — increases lifespan.

Conscientiousness. It's a personality trait researchers associate with healthier behaviors, greater self-reported healthiness, and longevity. Researchers advocate public health interventions to increase individual conscientiousness as a way to improve health and reduce health care expenses.

Unfortunately, personality traits are difficult for us to change, especially when we don't acknowledge a problem with our personality in the first place.

The concepts of zombie viruses and zombie behaviors provide a unique strategy to focus our attention on unhealthy beliefs and behaviors. Zombie virus eradication provides an intriguing mechanism by which we can increase our healthy beliefs, increase our healthy behaviors, increase our level of conscientiousness, and, ultimately, change our personality traits.

Annoying conscientiousness virus. This zombie virus makes us believe that healthiness can be taken too far. We believe that if conscientiousness is practiced all of the time, we'll never have any fun, we'll never be happy, we'll become less healthy, and we'll annoy everyone around us in the process. We believe it's somehow MORE healthy to occasionally do things that are UN-HEALTHY.

This virus gives us permission to disregard the health benefits of conscientiousness, or what TR refers to as the C word. It lets us ridicule the C word and hassle people who we think are health perfectionists and environmental perfectionists. It's another zombie virus endemic to Western society.

Anything but exercise virus. This zombie virus makes us willing to try anything our doctor suggests for health, short of exercise. It makes us consider exotic surgeries and medications. It infects our health care providers as well, making them offer surgery and medications to us rather than inspiring us to try harder with exercise.

High protein virus. This zombie virus makes us believe it's healthy to consume high protein beverages and foods. We think excess dietary protein helps us build muscle and bone even in the absence of exercise. We don't think about the risk of over-dosing on dietary protein and the risk of metabolic disorder, kidney stones, and tumor growth.

Quick-fix virus. This zombie virus makes us believe that high-tech medicine will someday provide a quick fix for aging. But, aging is not a disease. It is the side effect of increasing frailty in the body, which cannot be fixed by medications and surgeries. This virus discourages us from strengthening our fitness which is the only realistic treatment for aging.

CIRCADIAN FITNESS

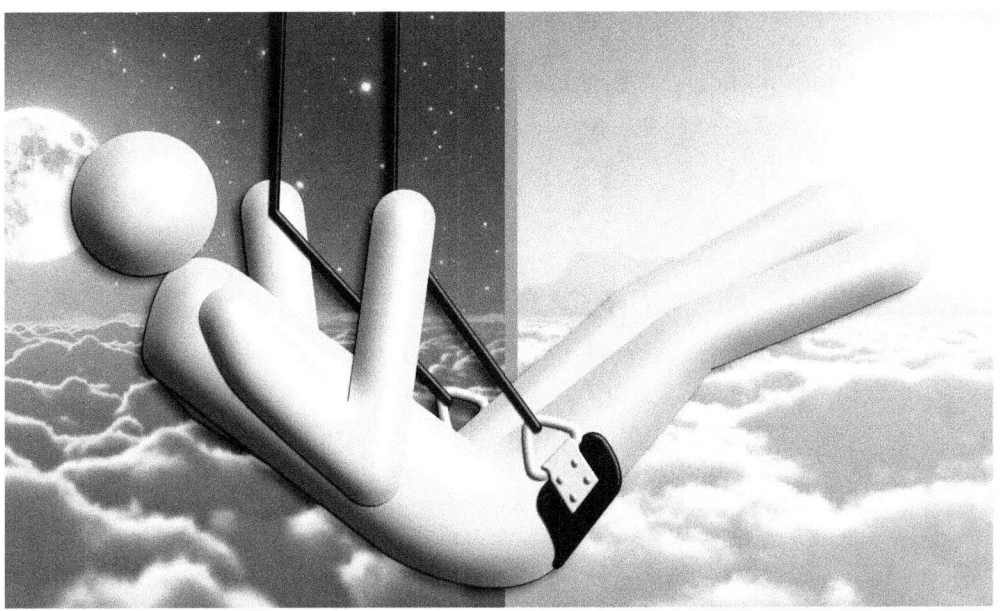

Circadian activity swings between deep sleep and full alertness.

We hear how sleep is important for our health. We hear how we're sleep deprived. We hear a lot of things about sleep that are hard to keep straight.

Circadian fitness helps us focus on the activities that must follow a 24-hour rhythm. Circadian fitness includes how many hours we sleep every night, how deep we sleep, and how well we adhere to a consistent sleep/wake schedule. Circadian fitness includes how well we adhere to a consistent meal and exercise schedule.

Circadian fitness is surprisingly important to total fitness. With neglect, our *Dimmer Switch of Circadian Fitness* shuts off, causing diseases such as Alzheimer's. With effort, we can pump our *Swing of Circadian Activity* and push our dimmer back up. We have evidence from the UCLA Alzheimer's study that we can not only delay Alzheimer's, we can reverse it.[**UCLA Study**]

In this chapter, we discuss the following topics:
- *From circadian fitness to frailty.*
- *What circadian fitness looks like.*
- *What circadian frailty looks like.*
- *Sleep length.*
- *Sleep depth.*
- *Sleep rhythm.*
- *Melatonin and DNA repair.*
- *Circadian fitness and us.*
- *Review.*
- *Imagine.*

FROM CIRCADIAN FITNESS TO FRAILTY

Circadian rhythm represents all the cellular processes inside the body that follow a 24-hour cycle. Our daily routine of sleeping, eating, and exercising influences the following circadian processes: management of alertness and drowsiness; removal of toxic metabolites from the brain; consolidation of memories and learning; synchronization of DNA repair in every cell; synchronization of gut microbial digestion; synchronization of energy storage and utilization; and rejuvenation of metabolic, microbial, immune, and mental fitness.[79]

Our circadian rhythm tends to fade so gradually, we lose track of how much we've lost and how much worse it can get. This slow fade is a problem, and TR wants to fix it.

TR has developed the concept of circadian fitness to help us see the big picture. Circadian FITNESS is based on the variation in circadian ACTIVITY, and is represented in the *Circadian Fitness and Activity Plot* below. If the concept and the plot work as designed, they should help us see where we are now and help motivate us to try harder.

The vertical axis on the plot represents circadian activity which describes the intensity of the circadian processes in the body. For convenience, we'll estimate it from our level of consciousness which varies from a low value when the mind is in deep sleep to a

---

79   Wikipedia. **Circadian_rhythm.** Accessed 2016. *en.wikipedia.org/ wiki/Circadian_rhythm*

high value when the mind is fully alert. But again, keep in mind that circadian activity represents ALL the sleeping, eating, and exercising schedules that must follow a 24-hour rhythm.

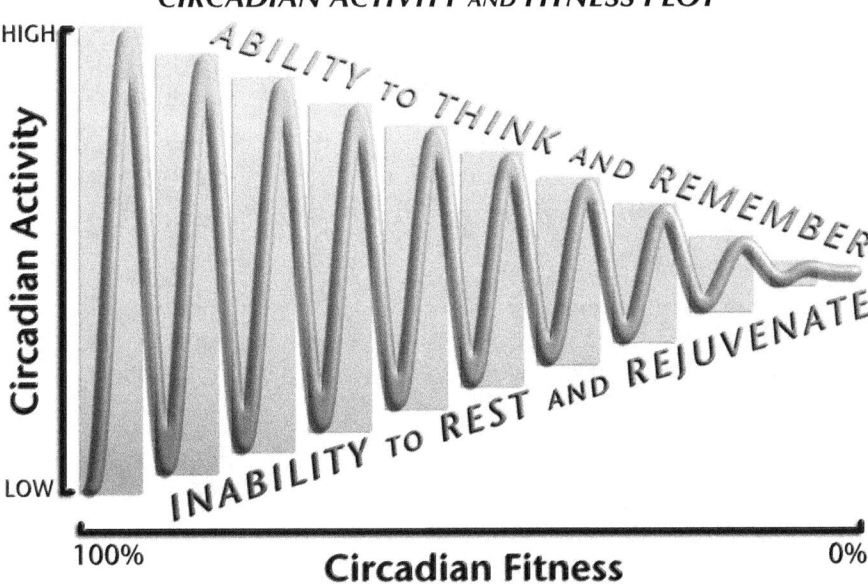

CIRCADIAN ACTIVITY AND FITNESS PLOT

The squiggly line on the plot can be imagined as the daily back and forth of the *Swing of Circadian Activity*. It swings from a state of rest and rejuvenation to a state of thinking and remembering. When we maintain our daily rhythm, our swing carves a wide path. When we neglect our daily rhythm, our swing etches a tiny path.

The horizontal axis represents circadian fitness. Fitness is highest when the daily back and forth of circadian activity is widest. At 100% fitness, the mind has the highest level of consciousness during the day and the deepest level of unconsciousness during deep sleep.

The vertical bars on the plot represent intervals of circadian fitness. Each bar can be imagined as a snapshot of the *Dimmer Switch of Circadian Fitness* that is slowly shutting off. We can push the dimmer higher by adhering to a schedule for sleeping, eating, and exercising.

The top edge of the plot represents the mind's fading ability to think and remember. The bottom edge of the plot represents the mind's increasing inability to rest and rejuvenate.

WHAT CIRCADIAN FITNESS LOOKS LIKE

In the *Circadian Fitness and Activity Plot* above, maximum circadian fitness is depicted by the tallest bar on the far left when the ABILITY to think and remember is maximum and the INABILITY to rest and rejuvenate is minimum.

Here are examples of what different levels of circadian fitness may look like.

%Fit	The Mind Can	Health Risks
100%	Sleep soundly all night, concentrate for long periods, and recall recent and past experiences.	None.
50%	Sleep lightly throughout the night, concentrate for shorter periods, and recall long-familiar experiences.	Increased risk for mental and metabolic disorders.
25%	Sleep in brief naps throughout the day and night, concentrate for short periods, and recall basic living skills.	Increased risk for dementia and metabolic disease.
1%	Drift in and out of sleep throughout the day and night.	Death.

WHAT CIRCADIAN FRAILTY LOOKS LIKE

In the *Circadian Fitness and Activity Plot* above, circadian frailty is depicted by the shortest bar on the far right. At this point, the body loses access to deep sleep and REM sleep. The mind cannot think, remember, rest, distinguish sleeping from wakefulness, or distinguish dreaming from reality.

Circadian frailty increases the risk of the following conditions:

Alzheimer's disease. Sleep disturbance decreases the clearance of toxic brain metabolites and increases the risk of Alzheimer's disease. Alzheimer's disease is the most common form of dementia. [80]

Mental frailty and metabolic frailty. Sleep disturbance increases the risk for daytime sleepiness, driving accidents, work-related accidents, depression, diabetes and liver disease. The most studied

---

80   Wikipedia. **Alzheimer's disease.** Accessed 2016. *en.wikipedia.org/ wiki/Alzheimer%27s_disease*

example of sleep disturbance is sleep apnea.[81]

SLEEP LENGTH

We've all been told to get eight hours of sleep every night. We've been told sleep is good and more is better. We've all become a little obsessed with getting eight or more hours of sleep at night.

It turns out the ideal amount of sleep is only seven hours. And if we skimp and get only six hours, it's not a big deal. Six hours is almost as good as seven hours.

Surprised? It gets even more surprising.

Eight hours of sleep appears to be TOO MUCH sleep. It increases our risk of premature death. Below is a plot of how mortality increases with eight or more hours of sleep. Anyone who sleeps nine or more hours per night is really pushing their luck with premature death. The following studies reveal that long sleepers are at increased risk of death, inflammation, and stroke.

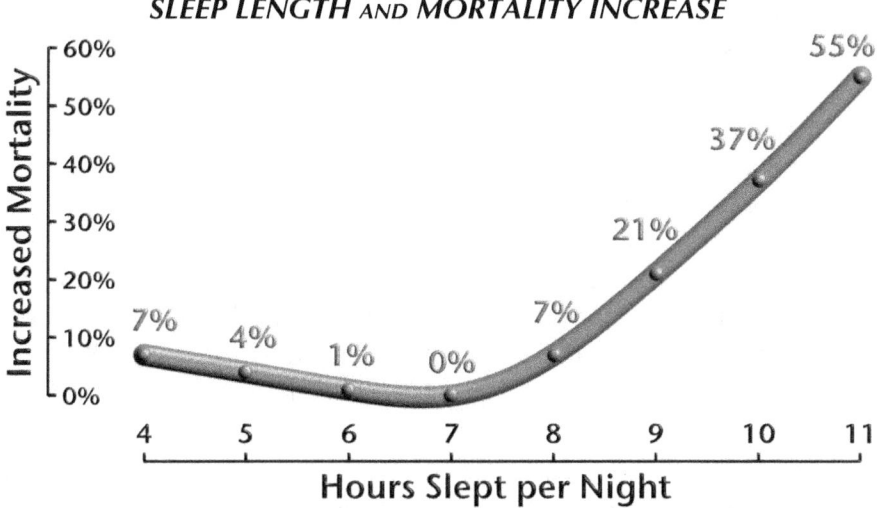

Sleep length and mortality increase. Chinese researchers construct the plot above based on a massive dataset of sleep length and mortality. They combine data from 35 research studies. The dataset includes 1.5 million subjects ages 40 to 83. The dataset spans ob-

81   Wikipedia. **Sleep apnea.** Accessed 2016. *en.wikipedia.org/wiki/ Sleep_apnea*

servation periods from 3 years to 25 years. The dataset includes 150,000 deaths during the various observation periods. The researchers compute the rate of mortality based on sleep length, and they discover that seven hours is the optimum.[82] The mortality data is plotted above.

The researchers discover that mortality follows a curve shaped like the letter J. The J curve is an important dose-response curve and will be discussed in more detail in *Book Two: Biological Happiness*. Shorter sleepers have a slightly increased mortality risk, but longer sleepers have a dramatically increased mortality risk. Too much of a good thing is a bad thing.

Sleep length and mortality increase for older adults. University of Pittsburgh researchers study the sleep length, inflammation status, and mortality of older adults. The researchers enroll nearly 3,000 adults around 74 years of age in their study. The researchers collect sleep length data and then monitor mortality over the next eight years.[83] The mortality data is plotted below. The plot has a similar trend as in the previous plot.

The University of Pittsburgh researchers confirm that seven hours is the optimum sleep length for older adults, like in the previous study. They also observe a J curve in the mortality trend, like in the previous study. The researchers observe that the shortest sleepers have a 30% increase in mortality, but the longest sleepers have a dramatic 49% increase in mortality. Again, too much of a good thing is a bad thing.

Sleep length and inflammation. UCLA researchers investigate how sleep length contributes to inflammation. The researcher pool data from 72 prior studies to create a dataset of over 50,000 study subjects. The researchers observe that long sleep associates with in-

82 Shen X, Wu Y, Zhang D. **Nighttime sleep duration, 24-hour sleep duration and risk of all-cause mortality among adults: a meta-analysis of prospective cohort studies.** Sci Rep. 2016 Feb 22;6:21480. *pubmed.gov/26900147*

83 Hall MH, Smagula SF, Boudreau RM, Ayonayon HN, Goldman SE, Harris TB, Naydeck BL, Rubin SM, Samuelsson L, Satterfield S, Stone KL, Visser M, Newman AB. **Association between sleep duration and mortality is mediated by markers of inflammation and health in older adults: the Health, Aging and Body Composition Study.** Sleep. 2015 Feb 1;38(2):189-95. *pubmed.gov/25348127*

creased blood markers for inflammation. Disturbed sleep also associates with increased inflammation. Short sleep does not associate with increased inflammation.[84]

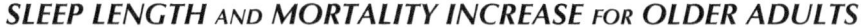

SLEEP LENGTH *AND* MORTALITY INCREASE *FOR* OLDER ADULTS

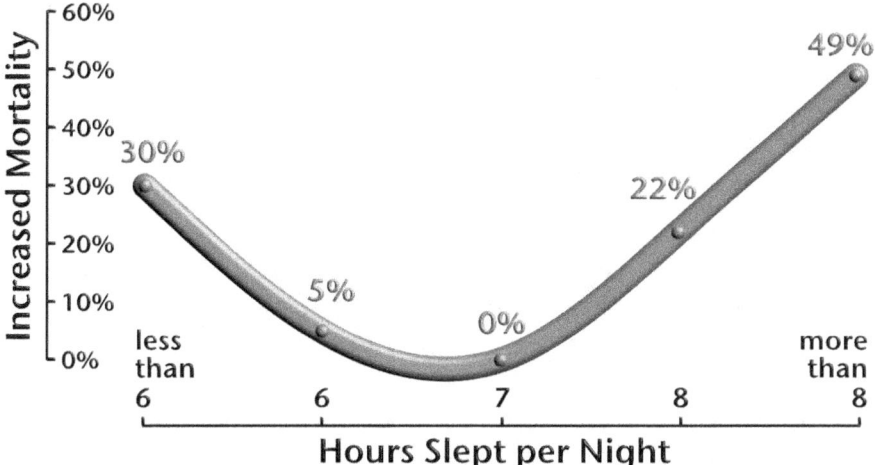

Hours Slept per Night

Sleep length and stroke risk. UK researchers investigate how sleep length contributes to the incidence of strokes. They first study the sleep length of nearly 10,000 adults ages 42 to 81 and monitor them for strokes for nearly 10 years. They observe a 46% increased incidence of strokes in the people who sleep more than eight hours, but an insignificant effect in the people who sleep less than six hours.[85]

The researchers perform a second study by pooling data from eleven prior studies to create a dataset of over 500,000 subjects. They observe that people who sleep more than eight hours have a 50% increased incidence of strokes.

84   Irwin MR, Olmstead R, Carroll JE. **Sleep Disturbance, Sleep Duration, and Inflammation: A Systematic Review and Meta-Analysis of Cohort Studies and Experimental Sleep Deprivation.** Biol Psychiatry. 2015 Jun 1. pii: S0006-3223(15)00437-0. *pubmed.gov/26140821*

85   Leng Y, Cappuccio FP, Wainwright NW, Surtees PG, Luben R, Brayne C, Khaw KT. **Sleep duration and risk of fatal and nonfatal stroke: a prospective study and meta-analysis.** Neurology. 2015 Mar 17;84(11):1072-9. *pubmed.gov/25716357*

Sleep depth is surprisingly important for circadian fitness. The most important aspects of sleep depth are deep sleep, REM sleep, and the hypnogram which plots them.

Deep sleep. It's called slow wave sleep. It's characterized by slow brain waves.[86] Researchers are only recently discovering what the brain is actually doing during deep sleep and why it is critical to circadian fitness.

During deep sleep, growth hormone is released into the body to coordinate tissue repair. This hormone rejuvenates metabolic fitness.

Most importantly, deep sleep is when the brain's circulatory system is most active.[87] It removes toxic waste products from the brain such as amyloid-beta and lipids. Deep sleep rejuvenates daytime alertness. Without deep sleep, the brain continues accumulating toxic waste products and loses daytime alertness.

The daytime accumulation of toxic waste products in the brain is consistent with sundowning syndrome. Dementia patients, including Alzheimer's patients, frequently display a daily relapse and remission in disease. Relapse occurs in the evening, or at sundown, and remission occurs in the morning after some quantity of deep sleep removes toxic waste products from the brain. Melatonin supplementation appears to encourage deeper sleep and ease the sundowning syndrome.[88]

REM sleep. It's also known as Rapid-Eye Movement sleep. It's characterized by random movements of the eyes and vivid dreams. It consolidates memories and reinforces daily learning. REM sleep rejuvenates mental fitness.[89]

Hypnogram. The depth of sleep over the course of a night is

86   Wikipedia. **Slow-wave sleep.** Accessed 2016. *en.wikipedia.org/wiki/Slow-wave_sleep*

87   Wikipedia. **Glymphatic system.** Accessed 2016. *en.wikipedia.org/wiki/Glymphatic_system*

88   Wikipedia. **Sundowning.** Accessed 2016. *en.wikipedia.org/wiki/Sundowning*

89   Wikipedia. **Rapid eye movement sleep.** Accessed 2016. *en.wikipedia.org/wiki/Rapid_eye_movement_sleep*

plotted on a hypnogram by sleep researchers.[90] Three different hypnograms are depicted below in the chart titled *Hypnogram: Sleep Depth by Hour*. These hypnograms are excerpted from a textbook on sleep disorders.[91] They represent typical hypnograms observed for a 12-year-old youth, a 23-year-old adult, and a 70-year-old adult.

HYPNOGRAM: SLEEP DEPTH BY HOUR

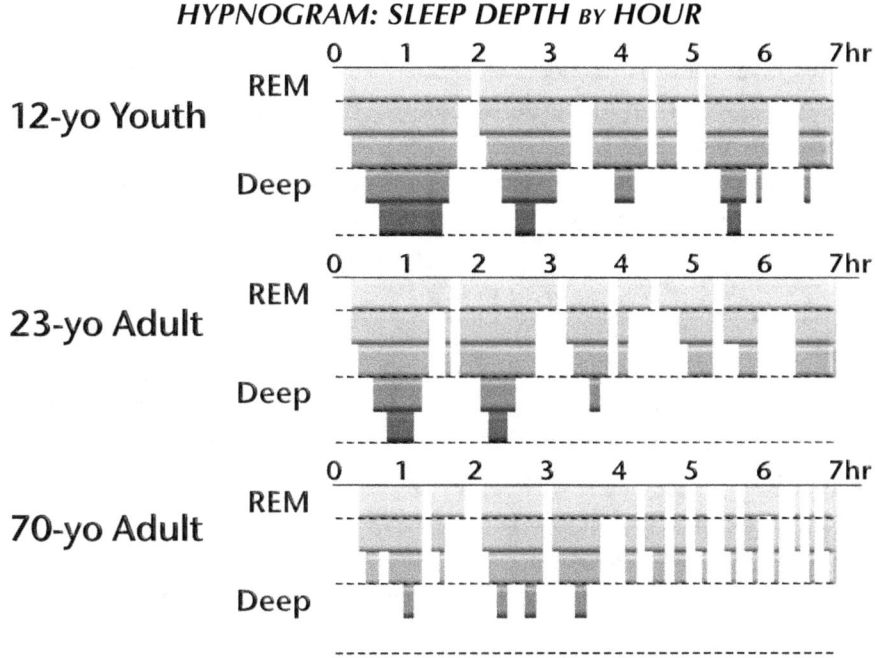

REM sleep is represented by the lightest shaded bar and diminishes with aging. Deep sleep is represented by the two darkest shaded bars and diminishes with aging.

Note how the hypnogram of the 70 year old is represented with a complete absence of the darkest shaded bar. These age-related changes in sleep are consistent with the following observations by sleep researchers.

Alzheimer's risk. Washington University Missouri researchers

---

90   Wikipedia. **Hypnogram.** Accessed 2016. *en.wikipedia.org/wiki/Hypnogram*

91   Figure created from data in Figure 2-7 on page 28 in Reite M, Weissberg MP, Ruddy J. **Clinical manual for evaluation and treatment of sleep disorders.** American Psychiatric Publications. 2009.

review how sleep disturbance contributes to Alzheimer's disease. Levels of amyloid-beta protein in the brain naturally increase during waking hours and decline during sleep. Amyloid-beta is flushed out of the brain during deep sleep when the brain's circulatory system is most active. If deep sleep is disturbed, amyloid-beta accumulates, aggregates, and forms plaques up to 20 years before the onset of dementia.[92]

Drug-induced deep sleep. University of Chicago researchers shows how increasing deep sleep causes an increase in growth hormone release. They dose eight healthy men with a drug that stimulates deep sleep, and they monitor the release of growth hormone as the men sleep. They observe a dose-response increase in deep sleep, and a dose-response increase in growth hormone release.[93]

Age-related hormone loss. The same team of University of Chicago researchers cnfirm age-related declines in deep sleep and REM sleep correspond to an age-related decline in GROWTH HORMONE. They study 149 healthy men — ages 16 to 83 years old. When they compare young adults to older adults: time spent in deep sleep drops from 20% to 5%; time spent in REM sleep drops from 20% to 10%; and daily growth hormone release drops from 600 micrograms to 100 micrograms.[94]

Age-related hormone loss. Brazilian researchers review how age-related changes in sleep lead to loss of muscle and frailty. They summarize how loss of rejuvenating sleep contributes to a loss of tissue repair hormones and a gain of tissue breakdown hormones. They single out the following hormones relevant to muscle loss: growth hormone, insulin-like growth factor-1, testosterone, cortisol,

---

92   Lucey BP, Bateman RJ. **Amyloid-beta diurnal pattern: possible role of sleep in Alzheimer's disease pathogenesis.** Neurobiol Aging. 2014 Sep;35 Suppl 2:S29-34. *pubmed.gov/24910393*

93   Van Cauter E, Plat L, Scharf MB, Leproult R, Cespedes S, L'Hermite-Balériaux M, Copinschi G. **Simultaneous stimulation of slow-wave sleep and growth hormone secretion by gamma-hydroxybutyrate in normal young Men.** J Clin Invest. 1997 Aug 1;100(3):745-53. *pubmed.gov/9239423*

94   Van Cauter E, Leproult R, Plat L. **Age-related changes in slow wave sleep and REM sleep and relationship with growth hormone and cortisol levels in healthy men.** JAMA. 2000 Aug 16;284(7):861-8. *pubmed.gov/10938176*

and insulin. They point out that: improvements in exercise, nutrition, and circadian rhythm promote health; but, treating patients with hormones directly has no effect.[95]

The research studies above confirm that sleep depth is an important factor in how circadian fitness preserves biological youth. And it confirms that the loss of sleep depth contributes to circadian frailty, metabolic frailty, and mental frailty.

SLEEP RHYTHM

Circadian fitness is strengthened by having a consistent sleep rhythm every single day of the week. It requires going to bed at the same time, waking up at the same time, and avoiding long daytime naps every single day — including weekends.

Researchers document how bad things get when we don't maintain a consistent sleep rhythm. They show that loss of rhythm causes circadian frailty, which then cascades into metabolic and microbial frailty.

Long daytime naps. Japanese researchers study how daytime napping contributes to cardiovascular disease. They pool the data from 11 previous studies to create a dataset of over 150,000 subjects who are monitored for over ten years. They group the subjects according to whether they nap and the length of their naps. They observe a J curve dose-response between the daily length of napping and the incidence of cardiovascular disease as shown in the plot below.[96]

The Japanese researchers observe napping between 15 and 30 minutes per day is associated with the lowest risk of cardiovascular disease. Avoiding naps or napping 45 minutes per day slightly increases risk by 5%. Napping 60 minutes per day increases risk by 20%. Napping 90 minutes per day increases risk by 50%. Napping

---

95 Piovezan RD, Abucham J, Dos Santos RV, Mello MT, Tufik S, Poyares D. **The impact of sleep on age-related sarcopenia: Possible connections and clinical implications.** Ageing Res Rev. 2015 Sep;23(Pt B):210-20. *pubmed.gov/26216211*

96 Yamada T, Hara K, Shojima N, Yamauchi T, Kadowaki T. **Daytime Napping and the Risk of Cardiovascular Disease and All-Cause Mortality: A Prospective Study and Dose-Response Meta-Analysis.** Sleep. 2015 Dec 1;38(12):1945-53. *pubmed.gov/26158892*

120 minutes per day increases risk by 95%.

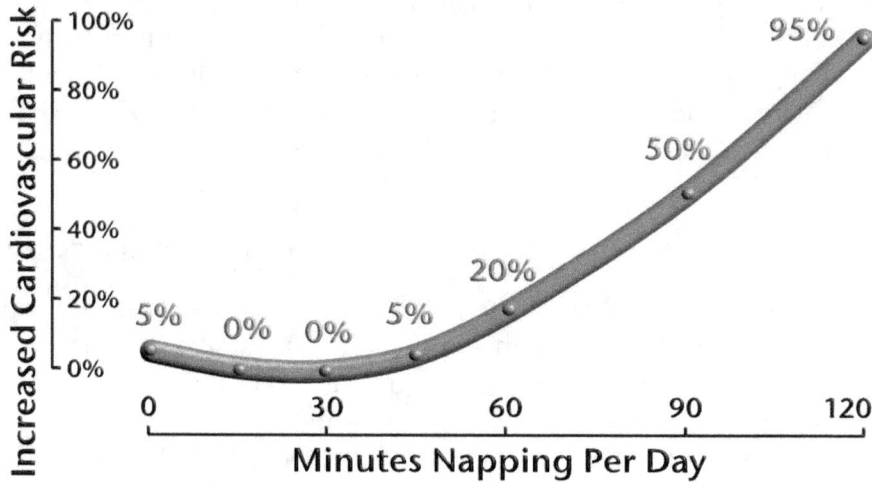

NAP LENGTH AND CARDIOVASCULAR DISEASE

Increased Cardiovascular Risk / Minutes Napping Per Day

The dose-response J curve observed with daytime nap length and cardiovascular disease is very similar to the J curve observed with nighttime sleep length and mortality. Once again, too much of a good thing is a bad thing.

Sleeping in. University of Pittsburgh researchers study how the disruption of circadian rhythm contributes to metabolic disorder. They study what happens when 447 healthy adults sleep later on weekends compared to weekdays. As circadian disruption increases, the researchers observe: lower levels of good cholesterol; higher triglycerides; higher fasting plasma insulin; insulin resistance; and adiposity.[97]

Inconsistent bedtime. Israeli researchers show how gut microbes have a circadian rhythm. The rhythm of the gut microbes is synchronized with the rhythm of the body. When the body's rhythm is disturbed, the gut microbes become unsynchronized, causing health disorder in the gut. Disruption of circadian rhythm causes dysbiosis — an overgrowth of bad microbes. Dysbiosis leads to inflammation and metabolic disorder.[98]

---

97   Wong PM, Hasler BP, Kamarck TW, Muldoon MF, Manuck SB. **Social Jetlag, Chronotype, and Cardiometabolic Risk.** J Clin Endocrinol Metab. 2015 Dec;100(12):4612-20. *pubmed.gov/26580236*

98   Thaiss CA, Zeevi D, Levy M, Zilberman-Schapira G, Suez J, Tengeler AC, Abramson L, Katz MN, Korem T, Zmora N, Kuperman Y, Biton I,

Gut microbes and dysbiosis will be examined in *Book Two: Biological Happiness.*

MELATONIN AND DNA REPAIR

Circadian fitness boosts melatonin levels in the body. When the eyes see complete darkness, the brain releases melatonin to the body.[99] Melatonin levels reach a maximum in the middle of the night, between midnight and two o'clock am.

Melatonin is often mistaken as a hormone that causes sleepiness. It's not. It's a hormone that SYNCHRONIZES circadian rhythm. It just happens that in human circadian rhythm, deep sleep is coordinated with peak melatonin levels. For nocturnal mammals, darkness still stimulates melatonin. In nocturnal circadian rhythm, full alertness is coordinated with peak melatonin levels. Melatonin is therefore not a sleep hormone; it's a circadian hormone.

Researchers have begun identifying the circadian effects synchronized by melatonin. Nearly every tissue in the body contains a receptor for melatonin.[100] When the melatonin receptor is stimulated by melatonin, the cell performs DNA repair. The nightly DNA repair strengthens genome stability and prevents cancer.[101]

With the invention of indoor lighting, computer screens, and electronic readers, the eyes are exposed to light in the evenings which suppresses melatonin levels and increases cancer risk. When

Gilad S, Harmelin A, Shapiro H, Halpern Z, Segal E, Elinav E. **Transkingdom control of microbiota diurnal oscillations promotes metabolic homeostasis.** Cell. 2014 Oct 23;159(3):514-29. *pubmed.gov/25417104*

99 Wikipedia. **Melatonin.** Accessed 2016. *en.wikipedia.org/wiki/Melatonin*

100 Poirel VJ, Cailotto C, Streicher D, Pévet P, Masson-Pévet M, Gauer F. **MT1 melatonin receptor mRNA tissular localization by PCR amplification.** Neuro Endocrinol Lett. 2003 Feb-Apr;24(1-2):33-8. *pubmed.gov/12743529*

101 deHaro D, Kines KJ, Sokolowski M, Dauchy RT, Streva VA, Hill SM, Hanifin JP, Brainard GC, Blask DE, Belancio VP. **Regulation of L1 expression and retrotransposition by melatonin and its receptor: implications for cancer risk associated with light exposure at night.** Nucleic Acids Res. 2014 Jul;42(12):7694-707. *pubmed.gov/24914052*

people work the nightshift and sleep during the daytime, their eyes may never see complete darkness. They suppress their melatonin levels and increase their cancer risk. Increasing age also suppresses melatonin levels and increases cancer risk.

A common way to improve circadian rhythm is oral supplementation of melatonin and tryptophan. Melatonin supplementation boosts circulating melatonin. Tryptophan supplementation boosts melatonin production and indirectly boosts circulating melatonin. [**102**]

Below is a review of recent research linking nightshift work and light at night to melatonin levels, metabolic frailty, and cancer risk.

Melatonin disruption. Tulane researchers present a compelling theory uniting circadian disruption with metabolic disorder and cancer. They discuss how melatonin synchronizes circadian rhythm throughout the body. Every tissue in the body must be synchronized to perform operations such as coordinating digestive function and initiating DNA repair. When the synchronization by melatonin declines; metabolism becomes unregulated, leading to metabolic disorder; and DNA repair becomes unregulated, leading to an accumulation of un-repaired DNA damage, genetic instability, and cancer. [**103**]

Nightshift work. German researchers review the evidence that circadian disruption increases cancer risk. They review 30 studies of flight personnel and nightshift workers. They compute a 40% to 70% increased risk of breast cancer for women and prostate cancer for men.[**104**]

E-books. Harvard researchers study how the use of modern tablets and e-books at night disturbs sleep and melatonin production. They study 12 healthy adults who read four hours before bed using an e-book or a printed book. They observe that e-books transmit more high-energy blue light into the eye than a passively lit

102 Wikipedia. **Tryptophan.** Accessed 2016. *en.wikipedia.org/wiki/Tryptophan*

103 Belancio VP, Blask DE, Deininger P, Hill SM, Jazwinski SM. **The aging clock and circadian control of metabolism and genome stability.** Front Genet. 2015 Jan 14;5:455. *pubmed.gov/25642238*

104 Erren TC, Pape HG, Reiter RJ, Piekarski C. **Chronodisruption and cancer.** Naturwissenschaften. 2008 May;95(5):367-82. *pubmed.gov/18196215*

printed book. They observe that e-books: reduce levels of melatonin; reduce nighttime sleepiness; shift circadian cycle later; and reduce morning alertness.[105]

CIRCADIAN FITNESS AND US

It should now be clear how important circadian fitness is to our youthfulness. It should also be clear how it depends on sleep length, sleep depth, and consistent sleep rhythm.

Sleep rhythm is hard for most of us to take seriously. On weekdays, we go to bed on time and wake up early. But on the weekend, we go to bed late to have a nightlife, or we wake up late to catch up on missed sleep. We don't realize how these indulgences have serious consequences.

We discussed earlier how strengthening the five fitnesses helps reverse the cognitive decline in early Alzheimer's patients.[UCLA Study] Alzheimer's disease may not seem like a disease we have to worry about when we're young. But we do. We can get it even when we're middle-aged. It's called early-onset dementia.

Prevalence. Indiana University researchers observe an increasing incidence of early-onset dementia starting at age 45. They estimate one in a thousand adults over age 45 has the condition. The researchers point to health risk factors that TR denotes as circadian frailty, metabolic frailty, and immune frailty.[106]

Risk factors. Dutch researchers notice that patients with early-onset dementia tend to have inconsistent sleep/wake rhythms and low levels of physical activity. They notice these patients tend to use anti-depressants and other medications that work on the brain.[107]

Mechanism. A UK researcher reviews all the ways sleep prob-

---

105 Chang AM, Aeschbach D, Duffy JF, Czeisler CA. **Evening use of light-emitting eReaders negatively affects sleep, circadian timing, and next-morning alertness.** Proc Natl Acad Sci U S A. 2015 Jan 27; 112(4):1232-7. *pubmed.gov/25535358*

106 Kuruppu DK, Matthews BR. **Young-onset dementia.** Semin Neurol. 2013 Sep;33(4):365-85. *pubmed.gov/24234358*

107 Hooghiemstra AM, Eggermont LH, Scheltens P, van der Flier WM, Scherder EJ. **The rest-activity rhythm and physical activity in early-onset dementia.** Alzheimer Dis Assoc Disord. 2015 Jan-Mar; 29(1):45-9. *pubmed.gov/24632989*

lems contribute to dementia. He reviews various mechanisms such as how lack of deep sleep allows amyloid-beta to accumulate, how melatonin deficiency correlates with dementia, and how inflammation contributes to brain degeneration.[108]

If you're beginning to see how we should take dementia and circadian fitness more seriously, then let's review the lifestyle behaviors that pump your *Swing of Circadian Activity* higher along with the ones that cause it to slow it down.

SWING OF CIRCADIAN ACTIVITY GUIDE

To Pump Higher:	To Slow Down:
Go to bed at the same time every weeknight and weekend night.	Stay up late on weeknights for work assignments or on weekends for "nightlife."
Sleep seven hours.	Sleep eight hours or more.
Get out of bed at the same time every weekday and weekend morning.	Get up early on weekdays and sleep in on weekends.
Avoid daytime naps. If a nap is necessary, keep it under 30 minutes.	Take long daytime naps of at least one hour.

This guide clarifies what you should and should NOT be doing to pump your swing and to keep your dimmer switch high.

And keep in mind, the four other fitnesses strengthen circadian fitness. For instance, regular exercise, regular meals, managing stress, and avoiding caffeine in the evenings strengthen deep sleep. [109]

Happy swinging.

108 Miller MA. **The Role of Sleep and Sleep Disorders in the Development, Diagnosis, and Management of Neurocognitive Disorders.** Front Neurol. 2015 Oct 23;6:224. *pubmed.gov/26557104*

109 Wikipedia. **Slow-wave sleep.** Accessed 2016. *en.wikipedia.org/wiki/ Slow-wave_sleep*

CHAPTER FIVE REVIEW

Circadian rhythm. It represents all the processes in the body that follow a 24-hour cycle. It includes alertness, drowsiness, removal of toxic metabolites from the brain, consolidation of memories, synchronization of DNA repair, synchronization of digestion, synchronization of energy storage and utilization, and rejuvenation of ALL FIVE fitnesses.

Sleep length. Seven hours of sleep every night is ideal for circadian fitness. The incidence of death increases slightly with six or fewer hours. The incidence of death increases dramatically with eight or more hours. The trend in mortality and circadian fitness can be visualized as a J-shaped curve in which seven hours is at the bottom of the letter J, six or fewer hours is on the low upward loop of the letter J, and eight or more hours is on the high straight side of the letter J.

Sleep depth. Deep sleep removes the daily accumulation of amyloid-beta protein in the brain. REM sleep consolidates the daily accumulation of learning and memories. We get the most deep sleep and REM sleep when circadian fitness is high.

Sleep rhythm. Going to bed at the same time every night, waking up at the same time every morning, and avoiding long naps helps synchronize sleep and helps synchronize digestion. Long daytime naps, light-emitting e-books, and inconsistent bed times and wake times cause circadian frailty which cascades into metabolic and microbial frailty.

Early-onset dementia. Researchers observe significant risk of dementia starting at age 45. They observe the following risk factors: poor sleep and wake rhythm, lack of exercise, low melatonin levels, inflammation, and use of anti-depressants and other medications that work on the brain.

CHAPTER FIVE IMAGINE

The growing market of fitness and sleep trackers suggests many people are becoming interested in fitness. These devices help gather activity data to monitor progress and provide inspiration. These devices arise from the personal awareness movement called Quantified Self.[110]

These devices — and the broader Quantified Self movement — are completely consistent with the concept of biological youth and the five fitnesses. We should look forward to the continued evolution of these devices, especially if TR inspires even more progress. It will be interesting to see if innovative device companies try to address all five fitnesses.

The fitness and sleep trackers are still in their infancy, which means they are most useful as motivational devices. They should never be used to diagnose a medical condition or a sleep disorder. They are not sufficiently reliable to replace the instrumentation used by clinicians and researchers to diagnose health disorders. They're designed for consumer convenience, not medical accuracy.

Sleep researchers cannot use sleep trackers to perform clinical research. They point out that deep sleep and REM sleep are defined by brain electrical activity and facial muscular activity. Currently available sleep trackers try to guess these activities by tracking heart rate, breath rate, and body motion. Some fitness trackers also try to guess sleep activity by tracking wrist motion, heart rate, skin temperature, and skin moisture.

WHEN SLEEP TRACKERS FAIL

The funniest example of how a sleep tracker can fail is contained in an online review.[111] The reviewer likes the particular tracker. It automatically detects when she's asleep. Other trackers require her to press a few buttons every night to clearly inform the tracker, "I'm going to sleep now."

Unfortunately, while the reviewer is working on her computer at her desk, she notices the fitness tracker thinks she's actually sleeping. Maybe it detected that her heart rate was low or her body temperature crossed below some threshold.

Such a mix-up would never happen in an actual sleep lab. A sleep lab is staffed by a technician who monitors the subject during the sleep analysis. A technician could easily distinguish a

---

110 Wikipedia. **Quantified Self.** Accessed 2016. *en.wikipedia.org/wiki/Quantified_Self*

111 LiveScience website. **Basis B1: Fitness Tracker Review.** Accessed 20-16. *livescience.com/42460-basis-b1-fitness-tracker-review.html*

subject lying flat on a bed from a subject sitting upright, working on a computer at a desk.

Fitness trackers cannot distinguish how a subject is positioned. It's a limitation that prevents researchers from taking these devices seriously.

For fun, we can imagine the mix-ups that may happen at a company that develops fitness trackers. Let's imagine how their sleep researchers test their tracker with a live customer.

"The heart rate and body temperature have crossed into the sleep range. The subject is now resting like a baby. We're looking good."

"I'm not asleep."

"Shushhhh... let's have some quiet. The sensors are in the sleep range. We're now collecting sleep data. We're looking good."

"Hey. It's me talking. I'm not asleep! I'm sitting here at my desk. I'm working on my computer. See? Watch me type on my keyboard." Clickety-click-click.

"Umm ... but your heart rate and your body temperature are very clearly in the sleep range. Please proceed with your nap and we'll keep collecting data. We're looking good."

"But I'm seriously not asleep. Would you please stop collecting data? I'm in full control of my hands. Watch this. I can type on my keyboard. I can even type an email to your boss right now. I'm telling him that ... this ... sleep ... and ... fitness ... tracker ... needs ... more ... work. Send!"

BIOLOGICAL AGE

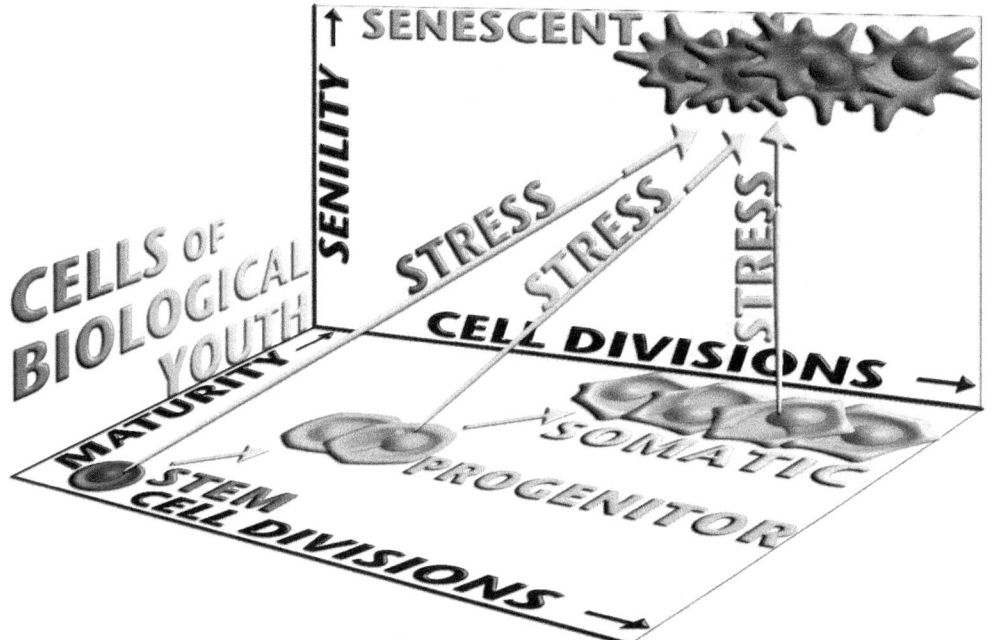

The journey to recovery supports the cells of biological youth.

Our bodies use stem cells to replenish the ecosystem of cells that make up our heart, brain, skin, and every other part of our bodies. But stem cells are only part of the story. Stem cells are child-like and must mature into teenager-like progenitor cells and then into young adult-like somatic cells. Our bodies depend on stem cells to replenish this team of cells — the Cells of Biological Youth.

The cells on this team are vulnerable to stresses caused by our lifestyles. Overwhelming stresses cause any cell of biological youth to leave the team and become a senescent cell.

Senescent cells are senile and curmudgeon-like. They stress their neighbor cells with inflammation and oxidation factors. Senescent cells act like tiny stress amplifiers. They form as a result of stress in the cell ecosystem. And once they form, they cause more stress in the ecosystem.

Our lifestyle preserves biological youth when it reduces stresses on our cell ecosystem. With less stress, our bodies have time to remove curmudgeonly senescent cells from the ecosystem before they further damage it. Our bodies can then replace them with cells of biological youth.

Our lifestyle accelerates biological age when it increases stresses on our cell ecosystem. With more stress, our bodies do not have sufficient time to remove senescent cells and replace them with cells of biological youth. Senescent cells then initiate a chain reaction. They amplify the stresses in our cell ecosystem and create an ever-burgeoning population of senescent cells.

In this chapter, we examine the following topics:
- *Cell maturity versus senility.*
- *The cells of biological youth.*
- *The Hayflick limit.*
- *Hayflick stress.*
- *Cell age*
- *Human age.*
- *Aging of the cell and the body.*
- *Nurturing the stem cell.*
- *Harnessing the cells of biological youth.*
- *Review.*

Advisory. This chapter is partly intended to inspire researchers to study cell aging and biological aging. To this end, it gets more technical than other chapters, but don't let it discourage you. Feel free to skim over the technical parts. And, the key findings will be presented again in the next chapter in a more humorous and less technical format.

CELL MATURITY VERSUS SENILITY

To understand how biological age happens, we must understand how our cells get old. There are two ways: cells can get more mature, which is usually a good thing, or they can get senile, which is usually a bad thing.

To make sense of cell maturity versus senility, we have to understand a few details about the stem cell niche, how cells divide, how they differentiate to become mature, and how they senesce to become senile.

Stem cell niche. It's the anatomic structure in body tissues that shelters stem cells from the larger ecosystem. The niche shelters stem cells within a carefully controlled microenvironment.[112] The niche can be imagined as a nursery school built and supervised by somatic cells who serve as teachers. The stem cells are like children attending the nursery school.

Most of the time, the niche keeps its stem cells in a dormant, non-proliferative state. The dormant state helps prevent over-exuberant proliferation and benign tumor formation. The dormant state is like a prolonged nap time for the child-like stem cells. When the niche receives signals that additional cells are needed in the ecosystem, it stimulates the stem cells to proliferate. The proliferation signals are like a bell that signals the end of nap time.

Every tissue contains stem cell niches to support tissue growth and repair. The most prominent niche can be found at the base of every hair follicle. It contains the stem cells that generate all the cells that add to the growing strand of hair. As long as our hair is still growing, the niches and stem cells in our hair follicles are still working.

Cell division. It's the process of one cell dividing into two identical cells, or clones. In the adult body, a stem cell can perform an UNLIMITED number of cell divisions when it is located inside the stem cell niche and when the niche receives the proper signals. A progenitor cell can perform a LIMITED number of cell divisions when it is located inside its target tissue and when it receives the proper signals from the tissue.[113]

Cell differentiation. It's the process of cell maturation — or how an immature cell gradually acquires mature features that "differentiate" it from other specialized cells in the body.[114] Cell dif-

---

112 Wikipedia. **Stem-cell niche.** Accessed 2016. *en.wikipedia.org/wiki/Stem-cell_niche*

113 Wikipedia. **Cell division.** Accessed 2016. *en.wikipedia.org/wiki/Cell_division*

114 Wikipedia. **Cellular differentiation.** Accessed 2016. *en.wikipedia.org/*

ferentiation is a form of cell aging that is analogous to the programmed aging during child development — how a child transitions through adolescence and puberty and acquires the features of a mature young adult.

The child-like stem cell has the fewest features and is characterized as IMMATURE and UNDIFFERENTIATED. The young adult-like somatic cell has the most features and is characterized as MATURE and FULLY DIFFERENTIATED. It is estimated there are about 220 different specialized somatic cells throughout the cell ecosystem of the human body.

Cell differentiation is regulated by signals from the extracellular matrix, neighboring cells, and circulating cell differentiation factors.

Cell senescence. It's the process of a cell becoming senile — or how an overly stressed cell suddenly acquires terrible new features. [115] Senescence can happen to any cell in any state of maturation. It can happen to a stem, progenitor, or somatic cell. It's a form of cell aging caused by stress and is unrelated to the form of cell aging during cell differentiation. Cell differentiation is how a cell becomes a mature cell. Cell senescence is how a cell becomes an OLD AND SENILE cell.

When a cell become senescent, it changes shape, enlarges, increases its energy consumption, and secretes noxious factors. The noxious factors cause inflammation, oxidation, degradation, and remodeling of surrounding tissues.

Senescence is NOT part of cell differentiation. Senescence can occur to any stressed cell regardless of its state of differentiation. Senescence should be imagined as an additional dimension of cell aging that is INDEPENDENT of the dimension of cell differentiation.

Cell differentiation is driven by a GENETIC PROGRAM, but cell senescence is NOT. Senescence is driven by unforeseen ENVIRONMENTAL STRESSES on a cell. It's just like how child development is driven by a GENETIC PROGRAM with clearly defined yearly milestones, whereas adult aging is driven by unforeseen LIFESTYLE and ENVIRONMENTAL STRESSES.

With these biological concepts in hand, we are ready to exam-

wiki/Cellular_differentiation

115 Wikipedia. **Senescence>Cellular senescence.** Accessed 2016. *en. wikipedia.org/wiki/Senescence#Cellular_senescence*

ine how stem cells and senescent cells contribute to the ecosystem of cells and to biological youth and age.

THE CELLS OF BIOLOGICAL YOUTH

As a society, we need to stretch our imagination to consider how lifestyle CONTROLS our rate of biological aging. We have a sense that lifestyle contributes to either HEALTHY AGING by slowing it down or PREMATURE AGING by speeding it up.

We need to stretch our imagination further to consider how the stem cells already inside the body link lifestyle to aging. We already consider how lifestyle is critical to health. And, we're beginning to consider how stem cells are critical to health. We just need to start considering how lifestyle is critical to stem cells in the body.

Currently, when we think about stem cells, we think about high-tech medical breakthroughs. We don't think about lifestyle. Stem cells seem so powerful and high tech. Lifestyle seems so mediocre and mundane.

Total Recovery has a strategy to help us think about stem cells and lifestyle at the same time. Say hello to the cells of biological youth!

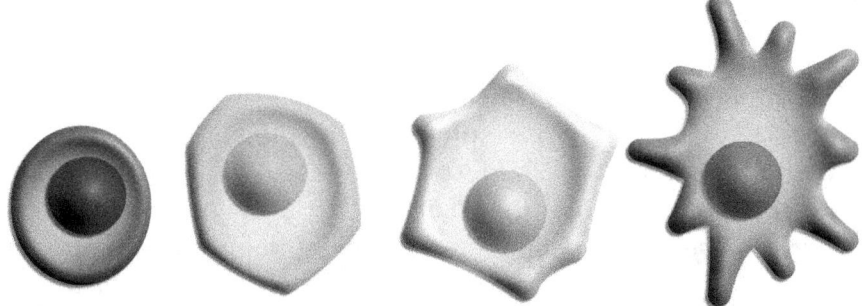

The stem, progenitor, somatic, and senescent cell.

STEM CELL.[116]
Undifferentiated state. It is like a child because it lacks features of a mature, fully differentiated cell.
Unlimited divisions. When it's in the stem cell nursery school AND it receives signals to activate, it can perform an unlimited number of

116 Wikipedia. **Adult stem cell.** Accessed 2016. *en.wikipedia.org/wiki/Adult_stem_cell*

cell divisions.

Unlimited lifespan. When it's in the stem cell nursery school, it has an unlimited lifespan.

Creates progenitor cells. When it leaves the stem cell nursery school, it differentiates into a progenitor cell.

Creates senescent cells. When overwhelmed with stress, it changes into a senescent cell.

PROGENITOR CELL.[117]

Partly differentiated state. It is like a teenager because it acquires the features needed to leave the stem cell nursery school. It seeks an apprenticeship. It joins a tissue that is welcoming new apprentices. It then enters a dormant state while awaiting signals from the tissue for when to start work.

Limited divisions. When it receives signals to activate, it can only perform a limited number of cell divisions to create clones.

Limited lifespan. When activated, it can only remain a teenager for a limited time.

Creates somatic cells. Its clones travel to their final work site within the tissue and differentiate further to become somatic cells.

Creates senescent cells. When overwhelmed with stress, it changes into a senescent cell.

SOMATIC CELL.[118]

Fully differentiated state. It is like a young adult because it has found its final location of employment. It is fully differentiated and has all the features it needs to support the surrounding tissue.

Limited divisions. It loses the ability to divide when fully mature.

Limited lifespan. It repairs itself every night to prevent the accumulation of daily wear-and-tear. When given sufficient time and resources for repair, it keeps itself running for a very long time.

Creates senescent cells. When overwhelmed with stress, it changes into a senescent cell.

---

117 Wikipedia. **Progenitor cell.** Accessed 2016. *en.wikipedia.org/wiki/Progenitor_cell*

118 Wikipedia. **Somatic cell.** Accessed 2016. *en.wikipedia.org/wiki/Somatic_cell*

Stressed state. It is like a senile curmudgeon because it stresses its neighbor cells, acquires terrible new features, and pollutes its neighborhood.

No divisions. It immediately disables its ability to copy its dna, so it cannot divide.

Unlimited lifespan. It slowly disables its kill switch, so it eventually becomes immortal.

Creates more senescent cells. It stresses neighboring cells so much that they may also become senescent. It cannot divide to create clones, but it converts neighbor cells to create more senescent cells.

Suppresses stem cells. It pollutes nearby stem cell niches. It stresses stem cells and causes them to differentiate and lose their capacity to divide.

Now that we've introduced the cells of biological youth, we can discuss the link between cell stress and the rate of biological aging. We can discuss how our lifestyle stresses our cells, causes them to become senescent, and causes the body to age. But first we have to clear up an important misconception about how cells get old.

THE HAYFLICK LIMIT

Skeptics of biological youth will argue that we cannot influence how long the cells in our body stay young. They'll argue that there's a limit on how long our cells can live and how many times our cells can divide.

The skeptics can thank Leonard Hayflick for their beliefs. He discovered the senescent cell in the 1960s. He convinced researchers that human cells have a limited lifespan. He convinced everyone that human cells can only divide a limited number of times before changing into a senescent cell. This limit became known as the HAYFLICK LIMIT. Much of the confusion about how our cells get old can be attributed to the Hayflick limit.

Back in the 1960s, researchers could only culture human can-

---

119 Nelson G, Wordsworth J, Wang C, Jurk D, Lawless C, Martin-Ruiz C, von Zglinicki T. **A senescent cell bystander effect: senescence-induced senescence.** Aging Cell. 2012 Apr;11(2):345-9. *pubmed.gov/ 22321662*

cer cells in the laboratory. They did not know how to culture healthy human cells. It was Hayflick who discovered how to keep healthy human cells growing and dividing in the laboratory.

Hayflick then embarked on a mission to dispel a popular notion that human cells could live forever.

Hayflick conditions. Hayflick pioneered cell culture conditions in the laboratory for human progenitor cells to grow and divide. Total Recovery denotes these laboratory conditions as Hayflick conditions. He cultured the progenitor cells to divide as many times as possible. He carefully counted the number of cell divisions, or population doublings.

Hayflick limit. After around 50 cell divisions, the progenitor cells stopped dividing. They appeared to reach a natural limit — that researchers now call the Hayflick limit. When Hayflick's progenitor cells stopped dividing, he described them as senescent.[120]

Hayflick proposed there must be a counting mechanism inside human cells to enforce the Hayflick limit. With further research, telomere caps at the end of each chromosome were identified as Hayflick counters. Telomere caps in progenitor cells tend to shorten with each cell division.[121]

Cancer bad, aging good. Hayflick pointed out that cancer cells have no Hayflick limit because they are immortal and can divide forever. He proposed that the Hayflick limit is be a safety mechanism to prevent progenitor cells from behaving like immortal cancer cells. He proposed that having progenitor cells turn into senescent cells is better than having them turn into cancer cells, so cell senescence is good. And he further proposed that the cells in our bodies turn into senescent cells as we get old, and because getting old is better than getting cancer, then aging is good.

Hayflick's limit and his theory of aging were not accepted at first. But Hayflick's conditions to culture progenitor cells were highly valuable and companies began selling equipment and reagents based on them. As more researchers used Hayflick conditions to culture progenitor cells, they confirmed that Hayflick conditions do indeed lead to a Hayflick limit. Researchers eventually came around

---

120 Wikipedia. **Hayflick limit.** Accessed 2016. *en.wikipedia.org/wiki/ Hayflick_limit*

121 Hayflick L. **How and why we age.** Exp Gerontol. 1998 Nov-Dec;33(7-8):639-53. *pubmed.gov/9951612*

to accept that aging is inevitable and there's not much we can do about it.

In hindsight, we know Hayflick was studying progenitor cells called fibroblasts and not stem cells.[122] Our understanding of the adult stem cell has changed since the 1960s. Now we know they exist. We know they're immortal. And we know they divide indefinitely — provided they're sheltered inside a healthy stem cell niche.

Given our current knowledge, we need to retire Hayflick's "cancer bad, aging good" dichotomy to the status of an outdated biological theory from the 1960s. We also need to retire Hayflick's benign characterization of the senescent cell. Now we know the senescent cell is a senile and curmudgeonly cell that stresses its neighbors.

HAYFLICK STRESS

In the past 20 years, we've learned that Hayflick conditions do not represent the conditions inside a healthy body. We've learned that Hayflick conditions cause stress to the laboratory cell. We've learned that cumulative stress causes a laboratory cell to become a senescent cell.

Hayflick made an important discovery with the senescent cell. He showed us how to create it from a progenitor cell in the laboratory, leading to groundbreaking discoveries about the senescent cell and about human aging.

In Hayflick's honor, Total Recovery denotes every stress that causes cell senescence as HAYFLICK STRESS. The following studies identify various sources of Hayflick stress caused by Hayflick conditions.

Growth factor stress. UK researchers demonstrate that culturing laboratory cells with serum growth factors causes cells to senesce. When they culture rat cells in serum-free media, the cells do not senesce.[123]

---

122   Wikipedia. **WI-38.** Accessed 2016. *en.wikipedia.org/wiki/WI-38*

123   Tang DG, Tokumoto YM, Apperly JA, Lloyd AC, Raff MC. **Lack of replicative senescence in cultured rat oligodendrocyte precursor cells.** Science. 2001 Feb 2;291(5505):868-71. *pubmed.gov/11157165*

Did you catch that? When rat cells are provided FEWER growth factors, they can be cultured FOREVER! Hayflick conditions include serum growth factors to stimulate cell growth. Therefore, growth factor stress is a Hayflick stress.

Atmospheric oxygen stress. Lawrence Berkeley National Lab researchers demonstrate that exposing laboratory cells to atmospheric oxygen pressure causes cells to senesce. Inside the body, the physiologic pressure of oxygen is ten-fold lower than atmospheric pressure. When they reduce the oxygen pressure from 21% (atmospheric) down to 3% (physiologic), they notice cultured mouse cells accumulate less DNA damage and do not senesce, even with growth factors present.[124]

Did you catch that? When mouse cells are provided PHYSIOLOGIC oxygen pressure, they can be cultured FOREVER! Hayflick conditions, however, provide ATMOSPHERIC oxygen pressure to laboratory cells, NOT PHYSIOLOGIC oxygen pressure. Providing laboratory cells physiologic oxygen pressure is more difficult, and researchers have a hard time justifying the extra work when Hayflick conditions are so convenient. But, working with cells at atmospheric oxygen pressure is like slicing an apple and noticing how the apple slices turn brown.

The slices weren't brown when they were inside the apple. The physiologic pressure of oxygen INSIDE the apple is much lower than the atmospheric pressure of oxygen OUTSIDE the apple. In the same way, cells INSIDE the body are comforted by physiologic oxygen. Cells brought OUTSIDE the body become stressed by atmospheric oxygen. It doesn't make sense to draw conclusions about how apples naturally age by inspecting apples that have been thinly sliced and exposed to air. The rapid browning of the thinly sliced apples is not natural aging, it is oxidation stress-induced aging.

Therefore, oxidation stress is a Hayflick stress. It's no wonder Hayflick's progenitor cells reached a Hayflick limit and became senescent cells. They were oxidizing like apple slices in front of his eyes.

Stem cell niche. Johns Hopkins researchers review how the

---

124   Parrinello S, Samper E, Krtolica A, Goldstein J, Melov S, Campisi J. **Oxygen sensitivity severely limits the replicative lifespan of murine fibroblasts.** Nat Cell Biol. 2003 Aug;5(8):741-7. *pubmed.gov/ 12855956*

stem cell niche creates a low oxygen environment for stem cells. Physiologic oxygen pressure can reach levels below 1%. Such an oxygen pressure is much less than the 21% atmospheric oxygen pressure of Hayflick conditions. Low oxygen pressure preserves the immortality of the stem cell in different tissues such as the embryo, bone marrow, and brain. The entire human brain maintains an oxygen pressure below 1% to preserve brain cells.[125]

Atmospheric oxygen causes DNA damage to the stem cell. Atmospheric oxygen causes the stem cell to differentiate into a mature cell and causes it to lose its unique ability to regenerate.

Stem cell confusion. A French researcher reviews how our understanding of the stem cell has been confused by Hayflick conditions in the laboratory. He reviews how most stem cell research in the laboratory is performed at ATMOSPHERIC oxygen pressure. This Hayflick condition causes the stem cell to behave unpredictably. When stem cell research in the laboratory is performed at PHYSIO-LOGIC oxygen pressure, the stem cell behaves in a profoundly different manner. He warns that most of our knowledge of the stem cell may need to be discarded.[126]

Researchers must be made aware of what atmospheric oxygen pressure is doing to their laboratory stem cells.

Human skin and hair. Human skin and hair are made of cells formed by cell division from stem cells under the skin[127] and inside the hair follicle.[128] The human body grows new skin and hair daily.

According to the Hayflick limit, skin stem cells should only be able to make 50 new layers of skin cells and will become exhausted within the first months of human life. According to the Hayflick limit, hair stem cells should only make hairs that are 50 cells long and

---

125 Mohyeldin A, Garzón-Muvdi T, Quiñones-Hinojosa A. **Oxygen in stem cell biology: a critical component of the stem cell niche.** Cell Stem Cell. 2010 Aug 6;7(2):150-61. *pubmed.gov/20682444*

126 Ivanovic Z. **Hypoxia or in situ normoxia: The stem cell paradigm.** J Cell Physiol. 2009 May;219(2):271-5. *pubmed.gov/19160417*

127 Wikipedia. **Stratum basale.** Accessed 2016. *en.wikipedia.org/wiki/Stratum_basale*

128 Wikipedia. **Hair follicle.** Accessed 2016. *en.wikipedia.org/wiki/Hair_follicle*

become exhausted within the first few weeks of human life. Such proposals are completely ludicrous. The Hayflick limit CANNOT apply to stem cells inside a healthy human body.

The Hayflick limit DOES apply to stem cells in a cancer patient receiving chemotherapy. Their stem cells typically become damaged by the chemotherapy, causing their hair to fall out. Cancer chemotherapy causes Hayflick stress inside the body. It causes cell senescence and will be discussed further in *Book Two: Biological Happiness*.

Based on this new research — and frankly, based on common sense — the human stem cell easily escapes the Hayflick limit when it is sheltered from Hayflick stress and Hayflick conditions. The human stem cell does not fit the Hayflick "cancer bad, aging good" dichotomy of cancer immortality versus cell senescence. It shows us there is a third option that's NOT CANCER and NOT AGING.

The third option means we don't have to be sour-pusses about how aging is inevitable, or how the Hayflick limit is inevitable, or how telomere shortening is inevitable.

The third option? Say hello to Total Recovery and the cells of biological youth!

CELL AGE

Researchers regularly invoke the Hayflick limit to explain how aging is inevitable. They invoke it despite the overwhelming evidence that the Hayflick limit is a laboratory artifact. We know cells can be cultured forever in alternative cell culture conditions. And we know human skin and hair stem cells continue dividing throughout our lifespan.

The Hayflick limit is based on the number of cell divisions. It traps everyone into thinking that the NUMBER OF CELL DIVISIONS represents the AGE OF THE CELL. It doesn't. It's a phenomenon that only occurs in Hayflick conditions.

The Hayflick limit and Hayflick conditions have become a snare for researchers. We have to fix this situation because we need researchers to study stem cells in the laboratory without aging the stem cells. Therefore, we need a different way to view the Hayflick limit, Hayflick stress, and Hayflick conditions. We need a breakthrough in imagination to understand what Hayflick ACTUALLY discovered.

Here's how Total Recovery gets us out of the trap of the Hayflick limit. There are two parts.

First, TR disentangles the concept of cell age from cell divisions by plotting cell age VERSUS cell divisions, which we'll do shortly. The image at the beginning of this chapter presents an artistic rendering of such a plot.

Second, TR quantifies the degree of association between cell age and cell divisions. In Hayflick's honor, TR denotes the degree of association as the HAYFLICK COEFFICIENT (C_H) which represents the magnitude of Hayflick stress on the cells.

The *Hayflick Coefficient Plot* below represents how cell culture conditions influence the aging of laboratory cells.

HAYFLICK COEFFICIENT PLOT

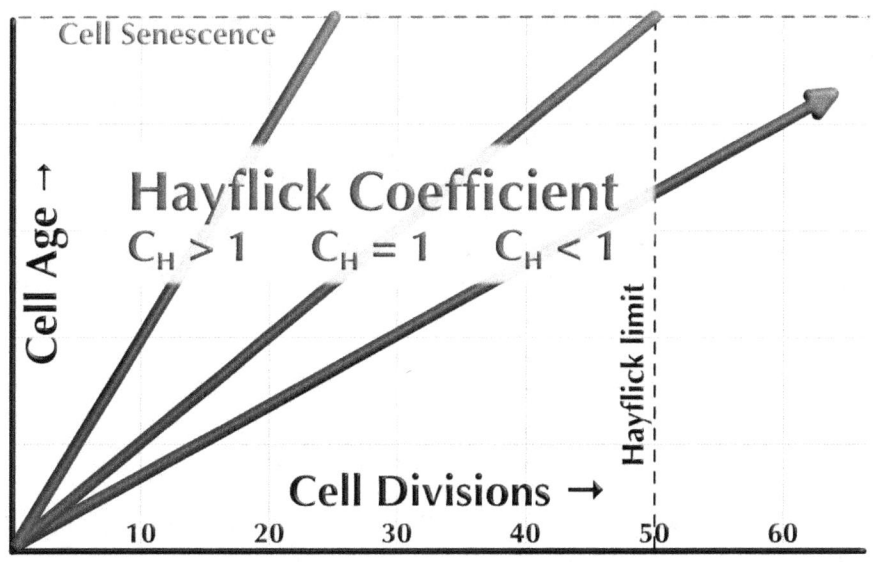

Value	Hayflick Stress	Cell Division Limit
$C_H > 1$	Higher	Shortened
$C_H = 1$	Typical	Typical
$C_H < 1$	Lower	Extended

In this plot, we use 50 cell divisions to represent the Hayflick limit, which is a typical value for human progenitor cells at atmospheric oxygen pressure.

The Hayflick coefficient (C_H) is computed from the cell division limit observed in Hayflick conditions compared to the cell division limit observed in alternative conditions. Both conditions would need to be evaluated by the researcher.

$$C_H = \frac{\text{Cell division limit in Hayflick conditions}}{\text{Cell division limit in alternative conditions}}$$

Typical stress. If alternative conditions provide an equivalent Hayflick stress, then the calculation of the Hayflick coefficient (C_H) may proceed as follows:

$$C_H = \frac{50 \text{ cell division limit in Hayflick conditions}}{50 \text{ cell division limit in alternative conditions}}$$

$C_H = 1$ represents typical Hayflick stress

Increased stress. If alternative conditions INCREASE Hayflick stress, then the calculation of the Hayflick coefficient (C_H) may proceed as follows:

$$C_H = \frac{50 \text{ cell division limit in Hayflick conditions}}{25 \text{ cell division limit in alternative conditions}}$$

$C_H = 2$ represents increased Hayflick stress.

Decreased stress. If alternative conditions DECREASE Hayflick stress, then the calculation of the Hayflick coefficient (C_H) may proceed as follows:

$$C_H = \frac{50 \text{ cell division limit in Hayflick conditions}}{100 \text{ cell division limit in alternative conditions}}$$

$C_H = \frac{1}{2}$ represents decreased Hayflick stress.

The Hayflick coefficient (C_H) and its plot allow us to escape the trap of the Hayflick limit. These concepts allow us to quantify the Hayflick stress on a cell in alternative cell culture conditions. These concepts provide a framework to test anti-aging interventions on laboratory cells — which is exciting.

HUMAN AGE

The concept that cell aging is inevitable ensnares us in another even bigger trap — the trap of human life expectancy. We're trapped into thinking that our current calendar age determines how many years we have left. We get our calendar age mixed up with our biological age. We don't realize how much lifestyle influences biological age.

Here's how TR gets us out of the trap of calendar age. There are two parts.

First, we disentangle biological age from calendar age by plotting them together on the same plot.

Second, we quantify the degree of association between biological age and calendar age. TR denotes the degree of association as the LIFESTYLE COEFFICIENT (C_L). It represents the magnitude of lifestyle stress on the body.

The *Lifestyle Coefficient Plot* below represents how lifestyle influences the aging of individuals.

LIFESTYLE COEFFICIENT PLOT

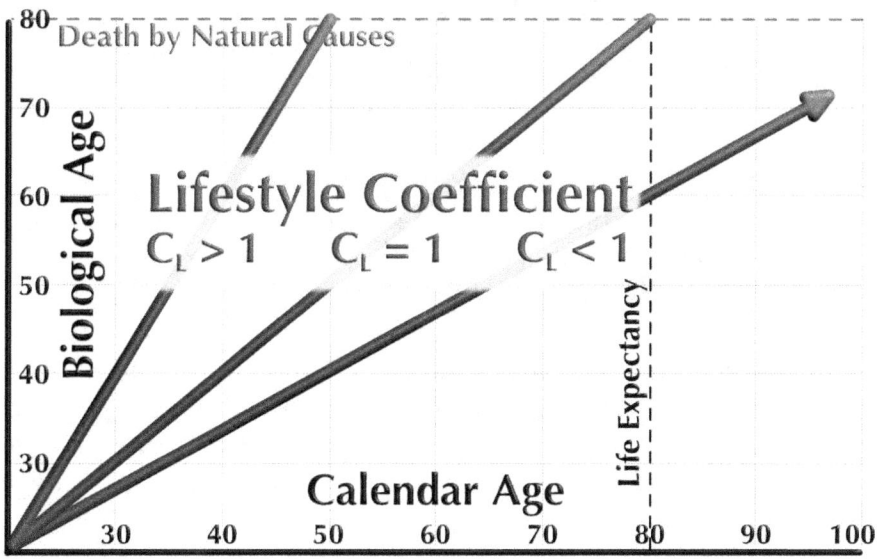

Value	Lifestyle Stress	Adult Lifespan
$C_L > 1$	Higher	Shortened
$C_L = 1$	Typical	Typical
$C_L < 1$	Lower	Extended

The *Lifestyle Coefficient Plot* should look like the *Hayflick Coefficient Plot*. It's because these processes are closely related. Cell senescence is what causes human age and death by natural causes. The senescent cell IS the natural cause of death. Therefore, the two plots are quite similar.

The lifestyle coefficient (C_L) is computed from the adult lifespan, which is the portion of the lifespan after age 20. We focus on the years from age 20 onward for the following reasons:

Childhood development represents aging that is hardwired. In other words, it is programmed into our genes. Adult aging from age 20 onward is strongly influenced by lifestyle and environmental stresses. In order words, it is NOT predetermined by our genes. The two forms of aging — childhood development and adult aging — are independent in the same way that the two forms of cellular aging — cell differentiation and cell senescence — are independent. In both cases, the second phase of aging — adult aging and cell senescence — is accelerated by stresses — either lifestyle stress or cell stress.

Did you catch that? The length of adulthood is a reflection of the tiny adulthoods of the many tiny cells in the body. Each cell in our body lives its adulthood according to the environment we create for it. When we provide a rewarding adulthood for our cells, they provide a rewarding adulthood for us.

The adult lifespan for the Western lifestyle can be estimated from life expectancy calculations provided by the CDC in a document called the National Vital Statistics Report.[129] In the 2010 report, the life expectancy at age 20 is 60 additional years, which is an average for all genders, races, and national origins of U.S. adults.

For any adult who dies of natural causes, their lifestyle coefficient (C_L) is computed from their particular adult lifespan resulting from their particular lifestyle, and it is compared to the average Western adult lifespan. Again, adult lifespan is the lifespan past age 20.

$$C_L = \frac{\text{Adult lifespan with Western lifestyle}}{\text{Adult lifespan with alternative lifestyle}}$$

Typical stresses. If a 20-year-old adult adopts the Western lifestyle, their lifestyle stress will typically lead to death by natural causes around calendar age 80. The calculation of lifestyle coefficient (C_L) would proceed as follows:

---

129 Arias, E. **United States Life Tables, 2010.** National Vital Statistics Reports. U.S. Centers for Disease Control and Prevention. U.S. National Center for Health Statistics. 2014. Volume 63, No 7. *cdc.gov/nchs/data/nvsr/nvsr63/nvsr63_07.pdf*

$$C_L = \frac{60 \text{ expected years past } 20}{60 \text{ observed years past } 20}$$

$C_L = 1$ represents typical lifestyle stress

Increased stresses. If a 20-year-old adult adopts an alternative lifestyle that INCREASES lifestyle stress, they could reach death by natural causes as early as calendar age 50. The calculation of lifestyle coefficient (C_L) would proceed as follows:

$$C_L = \frac{60 \text{ expected years past } 20}{30 \text{ observed years past } 20}$$

$C_L = 2$ represents high lifestyle stress.

Decreased stresses. If a 20-year-old adult adopts an alternative lifestyle that DECREASES lifestyle stress, they could reach death by natural causes as late as calendar age 110. The calculation of lifestyle coefficient (C_L) would proceed as follows:

$$C_L = \frac{60 \text{ expected years past } 20}{90 \text{ observed years past } 20}$$

$C_L = {}^2\!/_3$ represents low lifestyle stress.

The lifestyle coefficient (C_L) and its plot provide a way to quantify differences in lifestyle stress and adult lifespan. These concepts provide a framework to evaluate anti-aging interventions on adults — which is also exciting.

Typical values of the lifestyle coefficient (C_L)

We can estimate typical values of the lifestyle coefficient (C_L) for U.S. adults. We base it on data contained in the National Vital Statistics report published by the CDC. We use the following steps to process the CDC data:

1. We identify the cohort of U.S. adults who survive to age 20.
2. We divide the adult cohort into 10 equally populated groups according to total lifespan, from shortest to longest.
3. For each group, we estimate the average lifespan — using the median of the group to represent the average.
4. And for each group, we estimate the average lifestyle coefficient (C_L) — also using the median of the group.

The results are presented in the table below titled LIFESTYLE COEFFICIENT (C_L) ANALYSIS OF U.S. POPULATION. Curiously, the first three lifespan groups appear very different from the last seven groups. The first three groups have average lifespans spaced five to fifteen years apart. The last seven groups have average lifespans spaced three to four years apart.

LIFESTYLE COEFFICIENT ANALYSIS OF U.S. POPULATION

U.S. ADULTS GROUPED BY LIFESPAN	GROUP AVERAGE LIFESPAN	GROUP AVERAGE C_L
1	50	2
2	65	1.3
3	72	1.15
4	77	1.05
5	81	0.98
6	84	0.93
7	87	0.89
8	90	0.86
9	93	0.83
10	97	0.77

We can depict the aging of the 10 lifespan groups on the *Lifestyle Coefficient Plot of U.S. Population* below.

The first and last lifespan groups demonstrate the wide range of lifespans and lifestyle coefficient (C_L) values observed in the U.S. population.

Highest lifestyle stress. The first lifespan group represents 10% — or 1 in 10 — of U.S. adults who age the fastest. This group has survived to age 20 like the other nine groups. Yet this group only survives another 30 years and dies of natural causes around calendar age 50. This group ages at twice the rate of the average adult who typically survives 60 years past age 20. Therefore, this group has a lifestyle coefficient (C_L) of 2.0.

Lowest lifestyle stress. The last lifespan group represents 10% — or 1 in 10 — of U.S. adults who age the slowest. This group survives another 77 years past age 20, and dies of natural causes around calendar age 97. This group ages well below the rate for the average adult and has a lifestyle coefficient (C_L) of 0.77.

Infinitesimal lifestyle stress. There is a group of individuals, not shown on this plot, who live to calendar age 110, which is 90 years past age 20. The size of this group is very small, around 1 in 100,000 of U.S. adults.[130] This tiny group has a lifestyle coefficient (C_L) of $^2/_3$, or 0.67.

LIFESTYLE COEFFICIENT (C_L) PLOT OF U.S. POPULATION

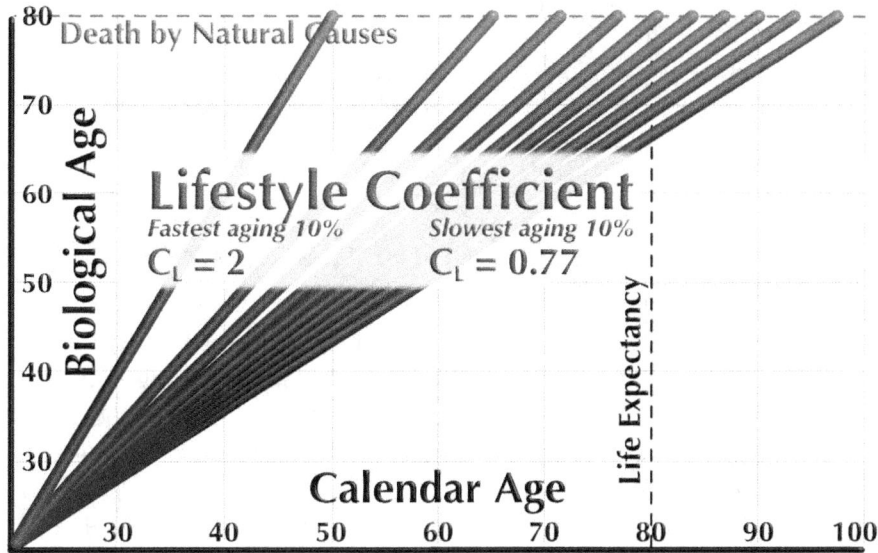

The striking differences in lifespans provide evidence for the range of lifestyle stress present in the U.S. population. It provides hope we may someday reduce lifestyle stress and reduce the aging of every group in the population.

Recent trends in lifestyle stress. U.S. researchers uncover startling recent trends in U.S. lifespan based on income and geography. They analyze 1.4 billion U.S. tax records and death records. Based on income, they observe lifespans for the top 5% have been increasing, but lifespans for the bottom 5% have been stagnant. Even worse, they observe lifespans for the bottom 5% have been eroding in some geographic regions.[131]

---

130 Andersen SL, Sebastiani P, Dworkis DA, Feldman L, Perls TT. **Health span approximates life span among many supercentenarians: compression of morbidity at the approximate limit of life span.** J Gerontol A Biol Sci Med Sci. 2012 Apr;67(4):395-405. *pubmed.gov/22219514*

131 Chetty R, Stepner M, Abraham S, Lin S, Scuderi B, Turner N, Bergeron A, Cutler D. **The Association Between Income and Life Expectancy in the United States, 2001-2014.** JAMA. 2016 Apr 10. *pubmed.gov/*

The U.S. researchers notice the following factors in regions with decreasing lifespans for the poor. lifestyle factors — more smoking, higher obesity, and less exercise; cultural factors — fewer immigrants and fewer college graduates; and government factors — lower government expenditures and lower home prices.

In the next section, we discuss ways the research community may help us monitor biological age at any calendar age. Such information would help us improve our lifestyles. Motivated individuals could optimize their lifestyles to decrease their lifestyle coefficients (C_L) and increase their lifespans.

AGING OF THE CELL AND THE BODY

The *Hayflick Coefficient Plot* and the *Lifestyle Coefficient Plot* allow us to ask big questions about aging. But researchers would have to run very long experiments to test the effects of modifying cell stress and lifestyle stress. Cell senescence can require up to six months of cell division in the laboratory. Death by natural causes requires an entire lifespan. We don't want to have to wait 50 or more years to find out whether some lifestyle factor increases or decreases lifestyle stress.

We need methods to monitor cell age and human biological age while the research subjects are still alive. We could run experiments over much shorter time periods and simply monitor ACTUAL changes in cell or human biological age. We could test interventions to SLOW cell or human biological aging.

Researchers are looking for methods to reliably measure cell and human biological age. We review the various proposals in the following studies:

PHYSIOLOGIC MEASURES. As discussed in *Chapter Two: Metabolic Fitness*, Duke University researchers use physiologic measures to estimate human biological age.[**Duke Study**] They derive a "Pace of aging" term that is equivalent to the lifestyle coefficient (C_L) over the 12 year span of their experiment. They observe values from near zero up to three. Their method would need to be adapted for cells in the laboratory.

Telomere. Telomere length is commonly used to measure cell and human biological age. The telomere is the structure that protects the ends of chromosomal DNA. It tends to erode with time and stress. However, University of Pittsburgh researchers point out that telomere length is so strongly influenced by gender and ethnicity that it ends up being an unreliable marker of age.[132]

Cell senescence. Spanish researchers review the many biomarkers of cell senescence.[133] These biomarkers indicate when a cell has become senescent. But these biomarkers cannot yet indicate how close a non-senescent cell is to becoming senescent, which would be a valuable indicator of cell age.

RNA expression. UK researchers use the RNA expression of genes to estimate human biological age.[134] This method could be adapted for cells in the laboratory.

Urine metabolites. German researchers use metabolites in urine to estimate human biological age.[135] This method could be adapted for cells in the laboratory by measuring metabolites in the growth medium.

Serum proteins. Swedish researchers use proteins in serum to estimate human biological age.[136] This method could be adapted for cells in the laboratory by measuring proteins secreted into the

132 Sanders JL, Newman AB. **Telomere length in epidemiology: a biomarker of aging, age-related disease, both, or neither?** Epidemiol Rev. 2013;35:112-31. *pubmed.gov/23302541*

133 Bernardes de Jesus B, Blasco MA. **Assessing cell and organ senescence biomarkers.** Circ Res. 2012 Jun 22;111(1):97-109. *pubmed. gov/22723221*

134 Sood S, Gallagher IJ, Lunnon K, Rullman E, Keohane A, Crossland H, Phillips BE, Cederholm T, Jensen T, van Loon LJ, Lannfelt L, Kraus WE, Atherton PJ, Howard R, Gustafsson T, Hodges A, Timmons JA. **A novel multi-tissue RNA diagnostic of healthy ageing relates to cognitive health status.** Genome Biol. 2015 Sep 7;16:185. *pubmed.gov/ 26343147*

135 Hertel J, Friedrich N, Wittfeld K, Pietzner M, Budde K, Van der Auwera S, Lohmann T, Teumer A, Voelzke H, Nauck M, Grabe HJ. **Measuring Biological Age via Metabonomics - the Metabolic Age-Score.** J Proteome Res. 2015 Dec 10. *pubmed.gov/26652958*

136 Enroth S, Enroth SB, Johansson Å, Gyllensten U. **Protein profiling reveals consequences of lifestyle choices on predicted biological aging.** Sci Rep. 2015 Dec 1;5:17282. *pubmed.gov/26619799*

growth medium.

Epigenetic regulation. UCSD researchers use the epigenetic regulation of DNA to estimate human biological age.[137] UCLA researchers also use epigenetic regulation of DNA to estimate human biological age.[138] Both groups show this method works for cells in the laboratory and cells in the body. The epigenetic method looks very promising.

If researchers have the means to measure cell age and human biological age, they could compute the Hayflick coefficient (C_H) and the lifestyle coefficient (C_L) with much shorter experiments. They would not need to grow and divide cells to the point of senescence or wait for adults to die from natural causes. They would speed up their studies dramatically.

But we need to adapt how we compute the Hayflick coefficient (C_H) and the lifestyle coefficient (C_L). Here are the revised formulas.

Hayflick Coefficient (C_H)

This quantity would be computed for a cell from its age at the current number of cell divisions when cultured in Hayflick conditions and when cultured separately in alternative conditions.

$$C_H = \frac{\text{Current cell age in alternative conditions}}{\text{Equivalent cell age in Hayflick conditions}}$$

Lifestyle Coefficient (C_L)

This quantity would be computed for a person directly from their current biological age and calendar age.

$$C_L = \frac{\text{Current biological age past 20}}{\text{Current calendar age past 20}}$$

---

137 Hannum G, Guinney J, Zhao L, Zhang L, Hughes G, Sadda S, Klotzle B, Bibikova M, Fan JB, Gao Y, Deconde R, Chen M, Rajapakse I, Friend S, Ideker T, Zhang K. **Genome-wide methylation profiles reveal quantitative views of human aging rates.** Mol Cell. 2013 Jan 24; 49(2):359-67. *pubmed.gov/23177740*

138 Lowe D, Horvath S, Raj K. **Epigenetic clock analyses of cellular senescence and ageing.** Oncotarget. 2016 Feb 14. *pubmed.gov/ 26885756*

These methods to compute the Hayflick coefficient (C_H) and the lifestyle coefficient (C_L) would enable researchers to run much shorter experiments and still gain valuable information about how cell stress and lifestyle stress influence aging.

NURTURING THE STEM CELL

Researchers are learning how the stem cell is sheltered in the stem cell niche and yet remains vulnerable to the health of the larger cell ecosystem. The extreme sensitivity of the stem cell to its surroundings is demonstrated in the following studies:

Youthful blood. Stanford researchers demonstrate how the age of blood determines the age of the stem cell. They swap the blood pumping from the heart of a young mouse with the blood pumping from the heart of an old mouse. The two mice remain strapped together while they constantly pump their blood into each other. The researchers observe the young blood rejuvenates stem cells in the old mouse to the youthfulness of stem cells in the young mouse. In other words, old blood makes stem cells old, and young blood makes them young.[139]

What makes old blood old? Senescent cells. They release inflammation and oxidation factors into the blood which pollute the cell ecosystem and stress the stem cells in the niches. When young blood is pumped into a mouse, the stem cells are no longer stressed by the pollution from senescent cells and suddenly become young again.

Stem cell niche. Taiwanese researchers review how the stem cell niche determines the age of the stem cell. They review the complex microenvironment that makes up the niche. They review how the niche is sensitive to the following factors: a high calorie diet damages the niche; and high or low vitamin D levels damage the niche.[140]

---

139 Conboy IM, Conboy MJ, Wagers AJ, Girma ER, Weissman IL, Rando TA. **Rejuvenation of aged progenitor cells by exposure to a young systemic environment.** Nature. 2005 Feb 17;433(7027):760-4. *pubmed.gov/15716955*

140 Wong TY, Solis MA, Chen YH, Huang LL. **Molecular mechanism of extrinsic factors affecting anti-aging of stem cells.** World J Stem Cells. 2015 Mar 26;7(2):512-20. *pubmed.gov/25815136*

Researchers are showing that when we nurture the niche, we nurture the stem cell. Their studies confirm the premise of this chapter: we can nurture the stem cell and the other cells of biological youth all by ourselves, and we can suppress the senescent cell all by ourselves. The Hayflick coefficient (C_H) should help promote the careful nurturing of the stem cell in the laboratory. A Hayflick coefficient (C_H) near zero would nurture stem cells to divide indefinitely. The lifestyle coefficient (C_L) should help promote the careful nurturing of the stem cell niches and the stem cells in our bodies. A lifestyle coefficient (C_L) near zero would nurture our stem cells to divide indefinitely.

FITNESS IN THE LABORATORY

The TR concept of the five fitnesses may provide new avenues for cell research IN THE LABORATORY. Researchers could assess whether their laboratory conditions promote stem, progenitor, somatic, or senescent cells by asking the following fitness-related questions:

Metabolic fitness. Can cells show evidence of nutrient excess, growth factor stress, oxidation stress, or other micro-environment stresses? Non-native cell-to-cell adhesion stress? Non-native sheer stress during liquid handling? Non-native radiation or UV stress? Can a tissue model with differentiated tendon or muscle cells show evidence of lack-of-use stress?

Immune fitness. Can cells show evidence of inflammation stress from dietary nanoparticles (e.g., titanium dioxide), environmental pollutants, restorative and cosmetic surgery materials, cosmetic piercing materials, and tattoo inks? Many cells activate an inflammasome if they detect foreign objects inside or outside the cell. [141] Are cells secreting inflammatory factors? What are the cells saying to each other with their secretions and surface proteins?

Microbial fitness. Can cells show evidence of exposure to microbial contaminants in laboratory materials? Researchers find many laboratory materials are sterilized, yet they're still contaminated

---

141 Wikipedia. **Inflammasome.** Accessed 2016. *en.wikipedia.org/wiki/Inflammasome*

with microbial products such as endotoxin.[142] Are cells exposed to viruses in laboratory materials? Do cells show evidence of the stress-induced reactivation of dormant DNA viruses? These viruses are called endogenous retroviruses[143] and transposable elements. [144]

Circadian fitness. Can cells show evidence of sufficient rest? Are cells maintaining synchronization of native clock signals inside the cells? Are cells receiving regular doses of melatonin? Melatonin is known to rise and fall in the body to coordinate cell rest and DNA repair.[145] Are cells maintaining native epigenetic marks such as DNA methylation, and chromosome structure marks such as histone methylation and acetylation?

HARNESSING THE CELLS OF BIOLOGICAL YOUTH

Our journey to recovery must harness the cells of biological youth as follows:

Child-like stem cell. We must strengthen metabolic fitness to nurture our nursery school-like stem cell niches in every body tissue to shelter our child-like stem cells. Our population of child-like stem cells must never be depleted or they will will no longer provide a steady supply of teenager-like progenitor cells to our tissues.

Teenager-like progenitor cell. We must strengthen total fitness to reduce the burden of tissue repair. Our population of teenager-like progenitor cells must never be depleted or they will no longer provide a steady supply of young adult-like somatic cells to our tissues.

---

142 Gnauck A, Lentle RG, Kruger MC. **The Limulus Amebocyte Lysate assay may be unsuitable for detecting endotoxin in blood of healthy female subjects.** J Immunol Methods. 2015 Jan;416:146-56. *pubmed. gov/25433222*

143 Wikipedia. **Endogenous retrovirus.** Accessed 2016. *en.wikipedia.org/ wiki/Endogenous_retrovirus*

144 Wikipedia. **Transposable element.** Accessed 2016. *en.wikipedia.org/ wiki/Transposable_element*

145 Wikipedia. **Melatonin.** Accessed 2016. *en.wikipedia.org/wiki/ Melatonin*

Adult-like somatic cell. We must strengthen circadian fitness to maximize nightly removal of toxic metabolites from the brain and to maximize the synchronization of DNA repair, digestion, energy storage, and energy utilization. Our population of adult-like somatic cells must be rested and refreshed every night, or they will no longer have a stress-free work environment every day.

Curmudgeon-like senescent cell. We must strengthen total fitness to minimize stresses on organs and tissues. Curmudgeon-like senescent cells must never reach a critical mass, or they will initiate a chain reaction of converting more cells in our tissues into senescent cells, and they will pollute our stem cell niches.

When our lifestyle strengthens the five fitnesses, it tips the balance to favor our health-promoting cells of biological youth. When our lifestyle causes unrelenting stress on our organs and tissues, it tips the balance to favor our polluting and stress-inducing senescent cells.

Circulating Progenitor Cells

Researchers are developing techniques to monitor the progenitor cells that circulate in the bloodstream. Researchers are demonstrating how these circulating cells contribute to our regenerative capacity, our resilience to disease, and our recovery from surgery. Researchers are demonstrating how our lifestyle can either promote these circulating cells or deplete them.

Here are a few key studies:

Progenitor depletion. Emory University researchers study how the depletion of circulating progenitor cells represents the loss of the regenerative capacity of the body. Cardiac patients with low levels of circulating progenitor cells display impaired regenerative capacity and are up to 250% more likely to die after heart surgery. Cardiac patients with high levels of progenitor cells display a high regenerative capacity and recover from their heart surgery more readily. [146]

---

146 Patel RS, Li Q, Ghasemzadeh N, Eapen DJ, Moss LD, Janjua AU, Manocha P, Al Kassem H, Veledar E, Samady H, Taylor WR, Zafari AM, Sperling L, Vaccarino V, Waller EK, Quyyumi AA. **Circulating CD34+ progenitor cells and risk of mortality in a population with coronary artery disease.** Circ Res. 2015 Jan 16;116(2):289-97. *pubmed.gov/25323857*

Lifestyle stress. Emory University researchers study how lifestyle stress exhausts stem cells and depletes the levels of circulating progenitor cells. People with increasing risk factors for heart disease — such as smoking, diabetes, hypertension and hyperlipidemia — show elevation of circulating progenitor cells when they're young but undergo stem cell exhaustion and show depletion of circulating progenitor cells as they age. On the other hand, people with no risk factors for heart disease show no exhaustion of stem cells and no depletion of circulating progenitor cells as they age.[147]

Lifestyle strength. Italian researchers review how regular physical exercise strengthens the stem cell niches, strengthens the stem cells, and sustains the levels of circulating progenitor cells. They review the mechanisms by which physical exercise boosts the production and longevity of circulating progenitor cells. They review how such boosts in circulating progenitor cells confer health benefits to people suffering from various cardiovascular diseases such as coronary artery disease (CAD), heart failure (HF), and peripheral artery disease (PAD).[148]

Therapeutic Stem Cells

We should not wait for future high-tech stem cell therapy. None of the proposed strategies under investigation addresses the loss of stem cell niches.

When a patient is in a state of low fitness, their body may have lost many of its functioning stem cell niches. Injecting therapeutic stem cells into such a person is like abandoning children on the mean streets of a big city with no adult supervision. Bad things can happen and will happen. Without the regulation imposed by the stem cell niche, therapeutic stem cells may proliferate and form benign tumors. Treatment efficacy may evaporate while long-term risk

---

147 Al Mheid I, Hayek SS, Ko YA, Akbik F, Li Q, Ghasemzadeh N, Martin G, Long Q, Hammadah M, Zafari AM, Vaccarino V, Waller EK, Quyyumi AA. **Age and Human Regenerative Capacity: Impact of Cardiovascular Risk Factors.** Circ Res. 2016 Jul 19. pii: CIRCRESAHA. 116.308461. *pubmed.gov/27436845*

148 De Biase C, De Rosa R, Luciano R, De Luca S, Capuano E, Trimarco B, Galasso G. **Effects of physical activity on endothelial progenitor cells (EPCs).** Front Physiol. 2014 Feb 3;4:414. *pubmed.gov/24550833*

of complications persists.

And, we should not subject ourselves to expensive stem cell therapies offered at private clinics. We must ask our physician if the necessary FDA approval has been obtained or if we will be part of an FDA-regulated clinical study.[149] Therapies provided outside of FDA regulation and without a multi-year follow up are dangerous.

Instead, we should strengthen the five fitnesses in order to support the cells of biological youth. When our lifestyle is therapeutic to our stem cell niches, our stem cell niches are therapeutic to our stem cells, and our stem cells are therapeutic to us. Naturally.

149 FDA.gov website. **FDA Warns About Stem Cell Claims.** Accessed 2016. U.S. Department of Health and Human Services. U.S. Food and Drug Adminstration. *www.fda.gov/forconsumers/consumerupdates/ucm286155.htm*

CHAPTER SIX REVIEW

Stem cell niche. This anatomical structure provides a sheltered and environmentally-controlled location (micro-environment) for stem cells. It is like a nursery school and the stem cells are like children. The niche is formed by somatic cells that are like the teachers of the nursery school. The niche keeps stem cells in a dormant state until it receives signals to stimulate the cells to proliferate. It exists in every organ and every tissue in the body.

Cell division. This process involves a stem cell or a progenitor cell dividing to make two identical cells. When a stem cell is inside a stem cell niche and is given signals to proliferate, it can divide an INFINITE number of times. When a progenitor cell is inside its target tissue and is given signals to proliferate, it can divide a LIMITED number of times.

Cell differentiation. This process involves an immature cell gradually acquiring mature features that "differentiate" it from other specialized cells. A stem cell differentiates into a progenitor cell, and a progenitor cell differentiates into a somatic cell. Cell differentiation is a form of cell aging — analogous to the aging during child development and maturation to young adulthood. It is regulated by the signals from the extracellular matrix, neighboring cells, and circulating cell differentiation factors.

Cell senescence. This process involves a stressed cell changing state and acquiring terrible new features. This process can happen to any cell in any state of differentiation — for example, a stem, progenitor, or somatic cell. A newly formed senescent cell changes shape, enlarges, increases energy consumption, and secretes noxious factors. The noxious factors cause inflammation, oxidation, degradation, and remodeling of surrounding tissues. Senescence is NOT part of cell differentiation. It is a form of cell aging completely INDEPENDENT from the form of cell aging during cell differentiation. It is caused by environmental stresses on the cell.

Stem cell. This cell remains undifferentiated and divides indefinitely when it resides in a stem cell niche. It is like a child and the niche is like a nursery school. Some stem cells are destined to leave the niche and differentiate to become progenitor cells. Stem cells can be placed under too much stress and change state to become senescent cells.

Progenitor cell. This cell is partly differentiated and divides a limited number of times when in its target tissue. It is like a teenager because it has just enough features to find its way from the stem cell niche to its location of residence in tissue. It remains dormant until it receives signals to become active and divide to form many clones. Its clones move to where new cells are needed, and they finish differentiation to become fully mature somatic cells. Progenitor cells can be placed under too much stress and change state to become senescent cells.

Somatic cell. This cell is fully differentiated and no longer divides. It is like an adult because it is located in its final place of employment in a tissue. It has all the mature features it needs to support the surrounding tissue. Somatic cells can be placed under too much stress and change state to become senescent cells.

Senescent cell. This cell can be formed from a cell in any state of differentiation after suffering overwhelming stress. It changes state and acquires terrible new features. It is like a senile curmudgeon because it stresses its neighbor cells and pollutes its neighborhood. It can stress its neighbor cells such that they become senescent cells too. It accumulates in the body with increasing biological age.

Hayflick conditions. This new term represents the 1960s-era laboratory conditions pioneered by Leonard Hayflick to culture human progenitor cells. Hayflick conditions cause progenitor cells to grow and divide up to a Hayflick limit and become senescent cells.

Hayflick stress. This new term represents the unfavorable stresses on laboratory cells exposed to Hayflick conditions. Hayflick stress induces cell aging and cell senescence. Researchers are finding new conditions to reduce the stresses on cells and to preserve the unique properties of stem cells.

Lifestyle stress. This new term represents the unfavorable stresses on the body caused by lifestyle and by the environment. Lifestyle stress induces cell aging and cell senescence inside the body which leads to biological aging.

Hayflick coefficient (C_H). This new term represents the magnitude of Hayflick stress on cells when cultured in any particular set of laboratory conditions. It is expressed relative to Hayflick conditions. The Hayflick coefficient (C_H) can be interpreted as follows:

Value	Hayflick Stress	Cell Division Limit
$C_H > 1$	Higher	Shortened
$C_H = 1$	Typical	Typical
$C_H < 1$	Lower	Extended

When a researcher measures the cell division limit for cells in Hayflick conditions and the cell division limit for cells in alternative conditions, the Hayflick coefficient (C_H) is computed as follows:

$$C_H = \frac{\text{Cell division limit in Hayflick conditions}}{\text{Cell division limit in alternative conditions}}$$

When a researcher measures the age of cells cultured in Hayflick conditions and the age of cells cultured in alternative conditions at the identical number of cell divisions, the Hayflick coefficient (C_H) is computed as follows:

$$C_H = \frac{\text{Current cell age in alternative conditions}}{\text{Equivalent cell age in Hayflick conditions}}$$

Lifestyle coefficient (C_L). This new term represents the magnitude of lifestyle stress on a person's body caused by their unique lifestyle and their unique environment. It is expressed relative to the Western lifestyle and environment. The lifestyle coefficient (C_L) can be interpreted as follows:

Value	Lifestyle Stress	Adult Lifespan
$C_L > 1$	Higher	Shortened
$C_L = 1$	Typical	Typical
$C_L < 1$	Lower	Extended

For any adult who dies of natural causes, their lifestyle coefficient (C_L) is computed from their particular adult lifespan past age 20, compared to the average Western adult lifespan as follows:

$$C_L = \frac{\text{Average adult lifespan with Western lifestyle}}{\text{Particular adult lifespan with unique lifestyle}}$$

For any adult with a known calendar age and a measured biological age, their lifestyle coefficient (C_L) is computed as follows:

$$C_L = \frac{\text{Current biological age past 20}}{\text{Current calendar age past 20}}$$

RECOVERY LIFESTYLE

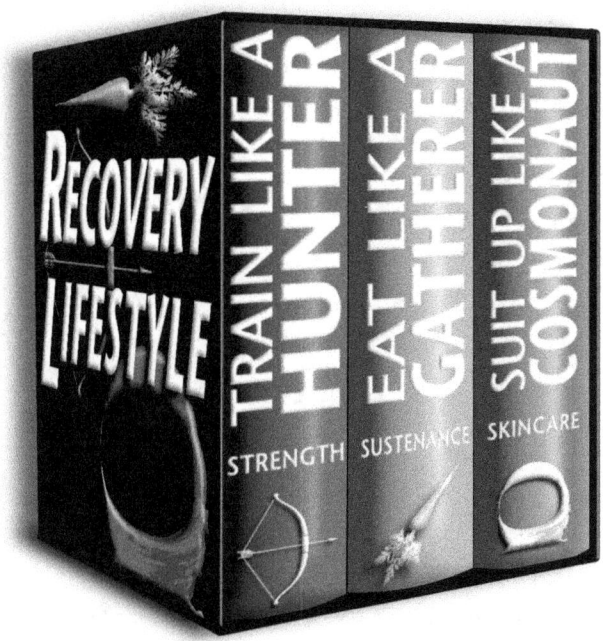

The journey to recovery follows the path of the recovery lifestyle.

Total Recovery is all about encouraging the recovery lifestyle — every concept, every metaphor, every visualization. The entire collection of TR books is designed to encourage the recovery lifestyle.

The recovery lifestyle preserves biological youth by strengthening the five fitnesses. It nurtures a recovery in the cell ecosystem in the body. It nurtures the stem cell and the other cells of biological youth. It prevents the senescent cell. It's based on equal parts research, imagination, and inspiration.

The recovery lifestyle is a collection of recovery behaviors that fall into three categories: STRENGTH, SUSTENANCE, and SKINCARE. Each category has an archetypal figure: the HUNTER, the GATHERER, and the COSMONAUT. The TR Series will eventually have an entire book dedicated to each category of recovery behaviors. The goal of this chapter is to get us started on our journey. The later books will add more color and detail.

In this chapter, we examine the following topics:
- *TR Strength.*
- *TR Sustenance.*
- *TR Skincare.*
- *Recovery lifestyle and the five fitnesses.*
- *The Escalator of Age.*
- *The Treadmill of Youth.*
- *Zombie years and dog years.*
- *The benefits of zombie years*
- *The clash of the zombies.*
- *Review.*
- *Imagine.*

TR STRENGTH

Train like a Hunter

The ancient hunter needed strength, endurance, and flexibility to capture prey and escape predators. Physical power was needed every day for survival. We need to train like a hunter every day for our survival too.

Training like a hunter is how we preserve metabolic fitness and the cells of biological youth. We discussed the importance of metabolic fitness in *Chapter Two: Metabolic Fitness*. Every day, we must pump the *Swing of Metabolic Activity*. When we keep our *Dimmer Switch of Metabolic Fitness* raised, we help strengthen the other four fitnesses.

But TRAINING like a hunter does not mean EATING like a hunter. The eating part comes in the next section.

Exercise is the most important thing we can do for our health. It's like taking a medicine that treats many diseases at once.[150] And, all its side effects are POSITIVE. It's a wonder drug.

People tell themselves they don't have the time for exercise — especially time for exercise every single day. But government statis-

---

150 Wikipedia. **Physical exercise.** Accessed 2016. *en.wikipedia.org/wiki/ Physical_exercise*

tics suggest the opposite is true.

Time survey. The U.S. Bureau of Labor Statistics publishes an annual survey of how adults divide their time among daily activities. The latest survey for calendar year 2015 shows that the busiest adults — adults between the ages of 20 and 65 — set aside only 15 minutes every day for recreation, sports, and exercise.[151] This figure includes the time of travel to and from recreation activities, which leaves VERY LITTLE time for exercise (if they even get any at all).

The survey also shows that these busiest adults set aside two hours and 30 minutes for watching television. This figure includes the time of travel to and from the couch, which leaves PLENTY of time to squeeze in some push-ups in front of the TV.

Training like a hunter is very different from lounging like a loafer. Yet the two activities are simple to combine.

Bodyweight exercise. TR Strength recommends BODYWEIGHT exercises — push-ups, pull-ups, planks, crunches, and sit-ups — that can be performed every day.[152] These exercises build strength utilizing the weight of the body. They can be performed at home or at work, so there's no time wasted driving to the gym. They can even be performed in front of the TV, which really eliminates all excuses.

Training like a hunter is only one notch more vigorous than current health recommendations. The Centers for Disease Control recommend strength training twice a week and vigorous aerobic exercise (such as running) one hour and 15 minutes every week.[153] By comparison, TR Strength recommends the following daily exercise: 15 minutes of bodyweight strength training; 15 minutes of running; and 15 minutes of stretching.

Recovering zombies should choose activities appropriate to

151 Bureau of Labor Statistics website. **American Time Use Survey.** Accessed 2016. U.S. Department of Labor. *www.bls.gov/news.release/ atus.toc.htm*

152 Wikipedia. **Bodyweight exercise.** Accessed 2016. *en.wikipedia.org/ wiki/Bodyweight_exercise*

153 CDC.gov. **CDC>Physical Activity>Physical Activity Basics>Adults.** Accessed 2016. Centers for Disease Control. U.S. Department of Health & Human Services. *www.cdc.gov/physicalactivity/basics/ adults/index.htm*

their current state of fitness. They should select activities to build strength, speed, endurance, flexibility, range of motion, and balance. If any activity causes soreness, they should take a rest from that particular activity until the soreness resolves. The point of TR Strength is to keep moving and stretching every day.

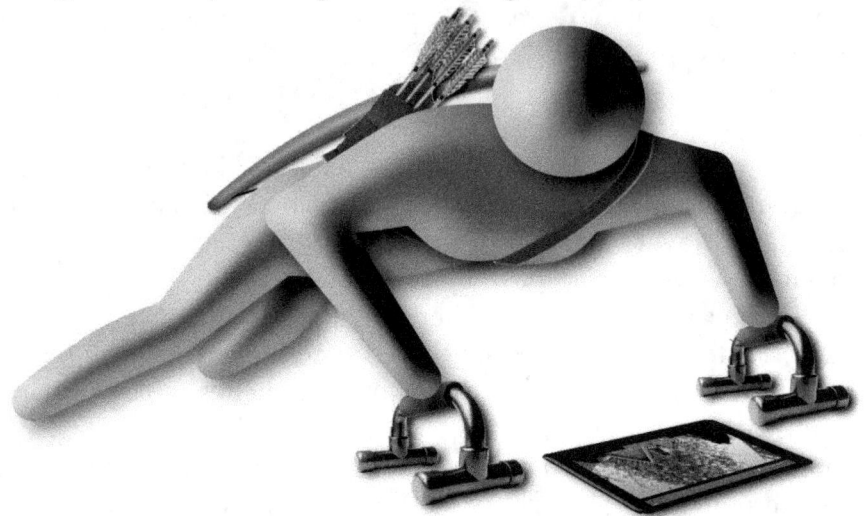

Bodyweight exercises eliminate all excuses.

Training like a hunter requires less than one hour of exercise every day. Paradoxically, this amount of exercise is small, but the health benefit is large, and yet we struggle to include it in our schedules. This triple paradox is at the heart of why TR is so much of a head game.

This part of the journey to recovery is guided by our decreasing desire to lounge like a loafer and our increasing desire for biological youth.

Sleep like a Hunter

The ancient hunter needed to hunt during daylight to catch prey and sleep during darkness to avoid nocturnal predators. TR Strength encourages us to sleep like a hunter, which means sticking to a regular circadian rhythm as if our survival depends on it.

We discussed the importance of circadian fitness in *Chapter Three: Circadian Fitness*. Circadian fitness strengthens microbial, immune, and mental fitness.

We pump our *Swing of Circadian Activity* by going to bed at the same time every night, sleeping seven hours every night, waking up at the same time every morning, and avoiding long daytime naps. When we keep our *Dimmer Switch of Circadian Activity* raised, we help strengthen the other four fitnesses.

This part of the journey to recovery is guided by our decreasing desire for nightlife and our increasing desire for biological youth.

TR SUSTENANCE

Eat like a Gatherer
The ancient gatherer needed wisdom to distinguish nourishing foods from poisonous foods. We need the same wisdom today to distinguish nourishing foods from snacks. TR Sustenance encourages us to eat like a gatherer with the Gatherer diet.

The Gatherer diet is like a Paleolithic version of the Vegetarian diet or like a Vegetarian version of the Paleolithic diet. It encourages the subset of foods that both diets come closest to agreement on. Here's how the food menus of the three diets overlap.

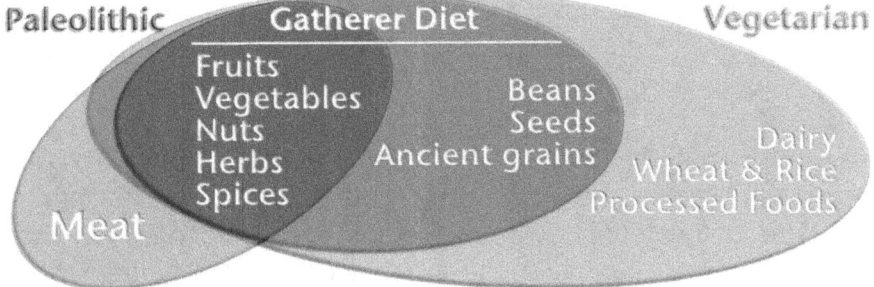

The menu of the Gatherer diet.

The Gatherer diet encourages foods low on the food chain with minimal processing. It encourages foods that research demonstrates are anti-inflammatory such as fruits, vegetables, nuts, beans, seeds, herbs, and spices.

The Gatherer diet discourages foods that are pro-inflammatory. Just like the Vegetarian diet, it steers away from meat. And just like the Paleolithic diet, it steers away from wheat gluten, refined carbs, processed foods, and dairy.

But there's a key difference between the Gatherer diet and the Paleolithic and Vegetarian diets. The Gatherer diet is NOT an exclusionary diet. It does not forbid or ban pro-inflammatory foods. It simply encourages nourishing foods and discourages everything else.

Another key difference is that the Gatherer diet is based on the best available research on nutrition and inflammation. The Gatherer menu is open to revision based on future research discovery. The food menu is not based on food doctrine, food orthodoxy, or food religion.

Anything that's not on the Gatherer menu is considered a snack. Recovering zombies can eat snacks as long as they eat nourishing foods first. In fact, newly recovering zombies should transition themselves gently to Gatherer foods. These foods are high in fiber and require gentle transition to allow time for the digestive system to adapt.

High fiber fruits, vegetables, seeds, and beans are needed to foster good bacteria in our gut. Our gut is colonized by over 1,000 species of bacteria, fungi, and archeae.[154] The good microbes are mutualistic, which means they help digest our food into valuable nutrients and fuel. Most microbes are commensal, which means they are harmless. Some microbes are pathogenic, which means they hurt us. High fiber foods support a diverse community of good gut microbes which helps prevent the growth of pathogenic gut microbes.[155]

This part of the journey to recovery is guided by our decreasing appetite for snacks and our increasing desire for biological youth.

The Gatherer diet will be presented in more detail in *Book Two: Biological Happiness* and in what will likely be *Book Three: Eat like a Gatherer*.

Cook like a Gatherer

The ancient gatherer ate foods raw while gathering and soaked and boiled foods when necessary. TR Sustenance encourages us to COOK like a gatherer, which means eating raw as often as possible. When cooking is desired, then stewing, steaming, and microwaving is recommended. Cooking like a gatherer is the most humble way to

---

154   Wikipedia. **Gut flora.** Accessed 2016. *en.wikipedia.org/wiki/Gut_flora*

155   Wikipedia. **Colonization resistance.** Accessed 2016. *en.wikipedia.org/wiki/Colonisation_resistance*

prepare food. It's also the most healthy.

The alternative to cooking like a gatherer is cooking like a hunter. This cooking method is very popular. Grilling, roasting, and baking food is celebrated in every restaurant, bakery, and backyard barbecue. Cooking like a hunter generates mouth-watering flavors in foods. Unfortunately, these mouth-watering flavors are seductively dangerous.

Exposing food to hot and dry cooking conditions causes chemical reactions inside food and creates a myriad of flavor, aroma, and browning molecules.[156] These new flavor molecules are chemically reactive, inflammatory, and carcinogenic. These flavor molecules bind to cellular receptors and trigger inflammation.[157] The cellular receptors for these flavor molecules exist on cells throughout the body, so inflammation increases everywhere in the body.

TR provides a guide to help gatherers visualize the full range of cooking choices. It's called the COOKING THERMOMETER OF INFLAMMATION and it's depicted below.

Cooking like a gatherer means using cooking methods at the low end of the thermometer. Such low temperature and high moisture cooking preserves the original flavors and aromas of foods without introducing the dangerous flavors from toasting and browning. Cooking this way preserves the inflammation-fighting and cancer-fighting powers of Gatherer foods.

On the other hand, cooking like a hunter means using cooking methods at the high end of the thermometer. Such high temperature and low moisture cooking introduces delicious but dangerous flavors, aromas, and browning of foods. Cooking this way exacerbates the inherently inflammatory effects of meat-based, dairy-based, and bread-based foods. Wood-fired pizza has got it all in one delicious but dangerous mouthful.

The Gatherer diet does not forbid or ban cooking like a hunter. Instead, it classifies the foods we cook this way as snacks. When we cook like a hunter, we're making snacks. We need to balance such snacks with nourishing foods cooked in a gatherer fashion. The more we eat AND cook like a gatherer, the more our overall diet is

156 Wikipedia. **Advanced glycation end-product.** Accessed 2016. *en. wikipedia.org/wiki/Advanced_glycation_end-product*

157 Wikipedia. **RAGE (receptor).** Accessed 2016. *en.wikipedia.org/wiki/ RAGE_(receptor)*

anti-inflammatory and anti-cancer.

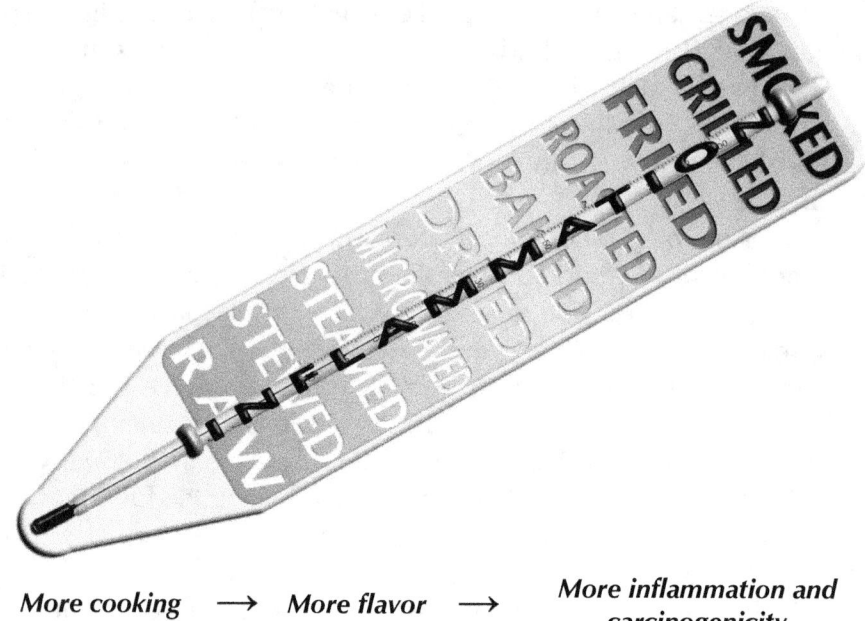

More cooking $\longrightarrow$ More flavor $\longrightarrow$ More inflammation and carcinogenicity

The Cooking Thermometer of Inflammation.

This part of the journey to recovery is guided by our decreasing appetite for cooking like a hunter and our increasing desire for biological youth.

Rest like a Gatherer

The ancient gatherer ate during daylight and fasted during darkness. TR Sustenance encourages us to REST like a gatherer, which means eating during the day and resting our metabolism during the evening and night.

Resting like a gatherer utilizes nightly fasting to pump the *Swing of Metabolic Activity*. There are many forms of intermittent fasting advocated in the literature and on the internet.[158] Many forms are based on alternating days of eating with days of fasting, which disrupts circadian rhythm. Nightly fasting is the only form that allows us to pump the *Swing of Metabolic Activity* AND the *Swing of Circadian Activity* at the same time.

If nightly fasting sounds awkward or unpleasant, please consid-

---

158 Wikipedia. **Intermittent fasting.** Accessed 2016. *en.wikipedia.org/ wiki/Intermittent_fasting*

er the following points:

Night eating. Going to bed with food in the stomach causes NUTRIENT STRESS while sleeping. The calories in the food exceed the body's low metabolic needs and stimulate unhealthy metabolism.[**159**] Nutrient stress stimulates fat storage. Even worse, it stimulates the partial burning of glucose which pollutes the body with incompletely burned fuel molecules.[**160**] It's like leaving the car idling in the garage all night with the door to the house open. The idling engine only partially burns fuel which pollutes the house with exhaust containing incompletely burned fuel vapor — carbon monoxide.

Night eating — especially consuming 25% or more daily calories after dinner — is associated with diabetes, obesity, depression, anxiety, and low self-esteem.[**161**]

Night fasting. Giving the stomach time to empty before going to bed reduces the nutrient stress on the body. Nutrient STRESS stimulates cells in the body to perform unnecessary growth and storage. Nutrient REST stimulates cells in the body to break down unnecessary or damaged cellular components and recycle them in a process called autophagy — a Greek word for self-eating.[**162**]

Autophagy is like patiently renovating an old house by stripping away damaged parts and replacing them with new parts.

Nutrient stress is like frenetically renovating an old house by patching over and covering up damaged parts with new parts and crossing your fingers that nothing serious goes wrong.

Breaking fast. Breakfast literally means to break the fasting peri-

---

159   Gallant A, Drapeau V, Allison KC, Tremblay A, Lambert M, O'Loughlin J, Lundgren JD. **Night eating behavior and metabolic heath in mothers and fathers enrolled in the QUALITY cohort study.** Eat Behav. 2014 Apr;15(2):186-91. *pubmed.gov/24854802*

160   Hood MM, Reutrakul S, Crowley SJ. **Night eating in patients with type 2 diabetes. Associations with glycemic control, eating patterns, sleep, and mood.** Appetite. 2014 Aug;79:91-6. *pubmed.gov/24751916*

161   Wikipedia. **Night eating syndrome.** Accessed 2016. *en.wikipedia.org/wiki/Night_eating_syndrome*

162   Wikipedia. **Autophagy.** Accessed 2016. *en.wikipedia.org/wiki/Autophagy*

od from the previous night.[163] The concept of nightly fasting has been around for a very long time. Breakfast is the most logical meal to break the fast. Breakfast eating is associated with more healthy blood lipids and heart rate.[164]

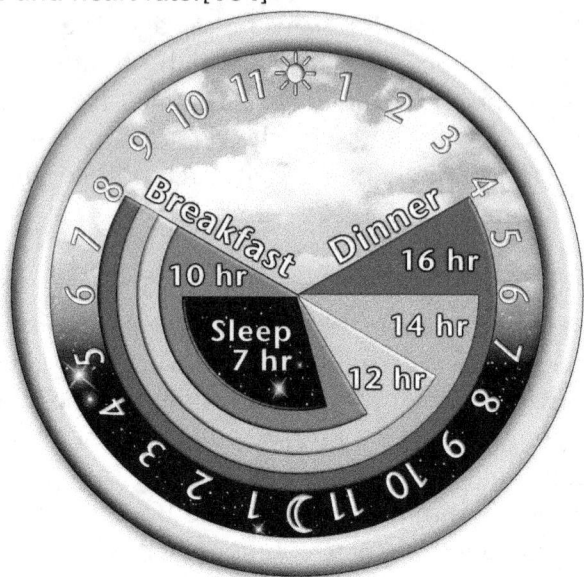

The Circadian Clock of Metabolic Rest.

NOT calorie restriction. Resting like a gatherer does NOT mean restricting calories. Yet, it confers the lifespan-boosting benefits of calorie restriction — WITHOUT calorie restriction.[165] A gatherer at rest is surprisingly happy, well-fed, and NOT hungry. It's the best of both worlds.

Stomach rest. Resting like a gatherer means we stop eating before bedtime to give the stomach time to finish digestion and enter a state of rest. The stomach typically needs a few hours to digest a

163 Wikipedia. **History of breakfast.** Accessed 2016. *en.wikipedia.org/ wiki/History_of_breakfast*

164 Yoshizaki T, Tada Y, Hida A, Sunami A, Yokoyama Y, Yasuda J, Nakai A, Togo F, Kawano Y. **Effects of feeding schedule changes on the circadian phase of the cardiac autonomic nervous system and serum lipid levels.** Eur J Appl Physiol. 2013 Oct;113(10):2603-11. *pubmed. gov/23922171*

165 Wikipedia. **Calorie restriction.** Accessed 2016. *en.wikipedia.org/ wiki/Calorie_restriction*

meal.[166] For example, eating breakfast at 8 am and finishing dinner by 8 pm provides a 12 hour period of eating and a 12 hour period of fasting. Falling asleep at 11 pm provides a three hour period of digestion before sleep.

Small intestine rest. Resting like a gatherer becomes more beneficial when we give our small intestine time to finish digestion and enter a state of rest. The transit time for a meal through the stomach and the small intestine can be as little as four hours and up to eight hours.[167] For example, eating breakfast at 8 am and finishing dinner by 4 pm provides an eight hour period of eating and a 16 hour period of fasting. Falling asleep at 11 pm provides a seven hour period of digestion before sleep.

Researchers use the terms NIGHTLY FASTING and TIME-RE-STRICTED FEEDING to describe what TR calls resting like a gatherer. Nightly fasting is demonstrating impressive health benefits in people and in laboratory animals.

Anti-Alzheimer's. The 36-point lifestyle intervention shown to reverse Alzheimer's symptoms (discussed in *Chapter Three: Circadian Fitness*) includes nightly fasting. Its nightly fast begins three hours before bedtime and runs 12 hours until breakfast.[168]

Anti-breast cancer. University of California San Diego researchers observe metabolic benefits of nightly fasting for women enrolled in a study of breast cancer risk. They observe improvements in blood sugar and glycated hemoglobin.[169] They observe improvements in blood markers of inflammation.[170] They ulti-

166　Wikipedia. **Stomach.** Accessed 2016. *en.wikipedia.org/wiki/Stomach*

167　Wikipedia. **Human_gastrointestinal_tract.** Accessed 2016. *en. wikipedia.org/wiki/Human_gastrointestinal_tract*

168　Bredesen DE. **Reversal of cognitive decline: a novel therapeutic program.** Aging (Albany NY). 2014 Sep;6(9):707-17. *pubmed.gov/ 25324467*

169　Marinac CR, Natarajan L, Sears DD, Gallo LC, Hartman SJ, Arredondo E, Patterson RE. **Prolonged Nightly Fasting and Breast Cancer Risk: Findings from NHANES (2009-2010).** Cancer Epidemiol Biomarkers Prev. 2015 May;24(5):783-9. *pubmed.gov/25896523*

170　Marinac CR, Sears DD, Natarajan L, Gallo LC, Breen CI, Patterson RE. **Frequency and Circadian Timing of Eating May Influence Biomarkers of Inflammation and Insulin Resistance Associated with Breast Cancer Risk.** PLoS One. 2015 Aug 25;10(8):e0136240. *pubmed.gov/*

mately observe a 26% reduction in the recurrence of breast cancer for women who fast nightly for 13 hours or more.[171]

Metabolic fitness. California State Los Angeles researchers review the metabolic benefits of time-restricted feeding. In humans and in laboratory animals, researchers observe improvements in the following metabolic parameters: body weight; blood fat levels such as total cholesterol, LDL cholesterol, HDL cholesterol, and triglycerides; blood sugar control such as glucose, insulin, and insulin sensitivity; and inflammation markers such as interleukin 6 and tumor necrosis factor-alpha.[172]

Resting like a gatherer does not require a specific number of hours of nightly fasting. It simply requires monitoring the hours of daytime eating and nighttime fasting. We can begin by reducing the size of our nighttime snack before bedtime. We can work on eliminating our nighttime snack so we have a three hour fast before bedtime. We can then start counting our nightly fasting time and increasing it up to 10 hours, then 12 hours, and so on.

This part of the journey to recovery is guided by our decreasing appetite for evening snacks and our increasing desire for biological youth.

TR SKINCARE

Suit-up like a Cosmonaut

The future cosmonaut will need diligent skincare to defend against toxic atmospheres on foreign planets and on an increasingly polluted Earth. TR Skincare encourages us to suit-up like a cosmonaut, which means diligent skincare to defend ourselves against ultraviolet radiation, oxidation, and dryness.

Suiting up is designed to keep us looking as YOUNG as possi-

26305095

171   Marinac CR, Nelson SH, Breen CI, Hartman SJ, Natarajan L, Pierce JP, Flatt SW, Sears DD, Patterson RE. **Prolonged Nightly Fasting and Breast Cancer Prognosis.** JAMA Oncol. 2016 Mar 31. *pubmed.gov/27032109*

172   Rothschild J, Hoddy KK, Jambazian P, Varady KA. **Time-restricted feeding and risk of metabolic disease: a review of human and animal studies.** Nutr Rev. 2014 May;72(5):308-18. *pubmed.gov/24739093*

ble for as LONG as possible. TR Skincare encourages a variety of strategies to protect our skin from wrinkling and our hair from from turning gray and falling out. While we nourish our skin with topical treatments on the outside, we use TR Strength and TR Sustenance to nourish the skin from the inside.

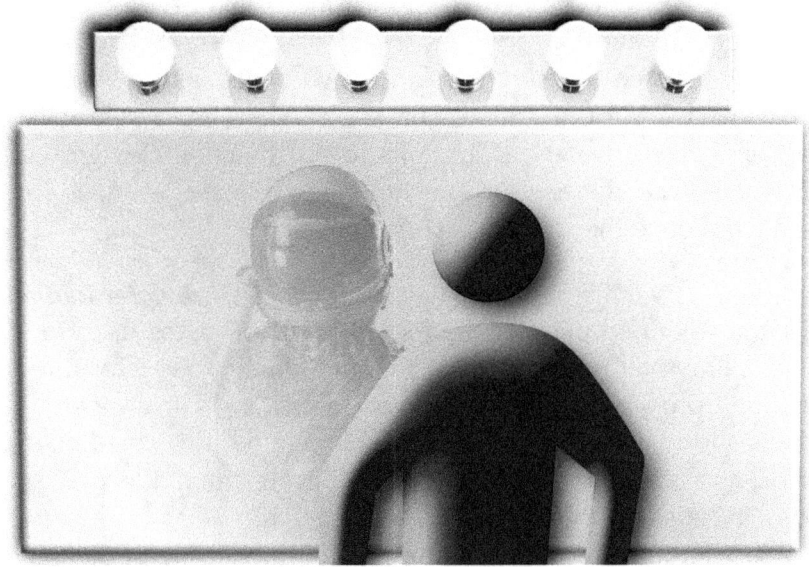

Suiting-up like a cosmonaut.

Our skin is the largest organ in our bodies.[**173**] It protects us from pathogens and from drying out. It warms us, cools us, and warns us about objects and conditions in our environment. The health of our skin supports the health of our bodies.

While our skin is our largest organ, the hair follicle within the skin is considered the smallest and most complex mini-organ in our bodies.[**174**] The hair follicle contains a stem cell niche that supports hair cell formation and hair growth. It contains an oil-secreting gland that helps moisturize and water-proof the skin. It contains a muscle that supports the stem cell niche and causes goosebumps. It contains a pigmentary unit that produces the pigment molecules

173 Wikipedia. **Human skin.** Accessed 2016. *en.wikipedia.org/wiki/ Human_skin*

174 Schneider MR, Schmidt-Ullrich R, Paus R. **The hair follicle as a dynamic miniorgan.** Curr Biol. 2009 Feb 10;19(3):R132-42. *pubmed. gov/19211055*

necessary for hair color.

The health of the hair follicle supports the health of the skin and the health of our bodies. Our hair protects us from UV exposure. Our hair protects us from cold. Our hair signals our state of internal health.

Suiting up reduces the stresses on the cells of biological youth inside our skin and hair follicles. Every day we shed old skin cells. Every day the stem cells in our skin grow new cells to replace them. Every time we cut our hair or shave our whiskers, we remove old hair cells. Every day the stem cells in our hair follicles grow new cells to replace them. Our skin and hair remain younger longer when we reduce the stresses on our stem cells.

Ultraviolet Radiation

For lighter-skinned people, the most significant stress on skin stem cells is ultraviolet radiation from sun and tanning bed exposure. UV radiation from any source causes photoaging and skin cancer.[175]

UV also causes vitamin D production in the skin, leading many zombies to believe that UV radiation is healthy. It's not. Once again, it causes photoaging and skin cancer. Mushrooms and dietary supplements provide vitamin D without causing photoaging or skin cancer. We must take UV exposure and vitamin D seriously by blocking one and getting the other by safer means.

Suiting up like a cosmonaut requires the following: minimizing direct UV exposure during the brightest hours of the day; covering skin and wearing sunglasses outdoors; and applying zinc oxide sunscreen EVERY morning of EVERY day. Sunscreen must be re-applied regularly. It must be applied whether its cloudy or sunny, cold or warm, or whether we're indoors or outdoors.

Inflammation, Oxidation, and Dehydration

The other stresses on stem cells are inflammation, oxidation, and dehydration. Inflammation is reduced when we support the balance of microbial communities on our skin and in our hair follicles. Topical essential oils boost the body's microbial and immune balances. Oxidation is reduced when we support the body's natural anti-oxidant defenses with TR Sustenance. Topical anti-oxidants boost the

---

175 Wikipedia. **Photoaging.** Accessed 2016. *en.wikipedia.org/wiki/ Photoaging*

body's anti-oxidant defenses. Dehydration is reduced when we support the body's natural oil production. Topical moisturizers boost the body's moisture defenses.

We need skin products to ease oxidation damage, wrinkles, and age spots. We need hair products to ease oxidation damage, gray hair, and receding hair. Unfortunately, the skin and hair products that claim to do these things seem too far-fetched, sketchy, or expensive.

Until such products become mainstream, we may consider making them ourselves. In the upcoming book on TR Skincare, we'll explore how to reduce inflammation, oxidation, and dehydration by adding natural osmoregulators[176], anti-oxidants, vitamins, amino acids, phytochemicals, and essential oils to lotions and hair products.

This part of the journey to recovery is guided by our decreasing neglect of skincare and our increasing desire for biological youth.

Prepare like a Cosmonaut

When suiting up, a cosmonaut prepares their body and the microbial population that lives on it. A cosmonaut views the body as a micro-planet with various microbial ecosystems ranging from tropical to desert-like. The cosmonaut prepares their body to nurture a diverse community of beneficial microbes and to suppress invasion by pathogenic microbes. TR Skincare encourages us to prepare like a cosmonaut which means cleaning our skin regularly and cleaning our teeth and gums after every meal.

Our skin is colonized by over 1,000 species of bacteria and over 80 species of fungi. Microbes can be beneficial, neutral, or pathogenic. Microbes alternate between these roles depending on the size of their population, where they are located, and whether they enter the bloodstream through an injury. Microbes compete with each other and keep each others' populations in check. A diverse community of microbes tends to suppress the invasion of pathogenic microbes.[177]

Because microbes feed on our dead skin cells, secreted oils,

---

176 Wikipedia. **Osmoregulation.** Accessed 2016. *en.wikipedia.org/wiki/Osmoregulation*

177 Wikipedia. **Skin flora.** Accessed 2016. *en.wikipedia.org/wiki/Skin_flora*

and secreted sweat, we must wash regularly to prevent excess build-up. But we must not wash too often or use harsh chemical detergents because we may damage our skin. We must not use anti-microbial soaps because we may cause imbalances in our microbial populations or breed antibiotic resistance.

Microbial imbalance leads to inflammation in the skin and hair follicles. Inflammation puts stress on the stem cells in our skin and our hair follicles and can lead to skin and hair disorder.[178] Inflammation can cause flaky skin, dandruff, roughness, itchiness, redness, facial acne, and hair loss.[179]

The mouth is colonized by many bacteria and fungi.[180] Because microbes feed on the sugars in our food, we must brush and floss regularly to prevent over-colonization. Tooth cavities and gum disease can lead to more serious internal diseases such as cardiac disease[181] and Alzheimer's disease.[182]

Anti-Alzheimer's. The 36-point lifestyle intervention shown to reverse the cognitive decline of Alzheimer's patients (discussed in *Chapter Three: Circadian Fitness*) includes brushing and flossing. Patients in the study are encouraged to try electric toothbrushes and water flossers.[**UCLA Study**]

This part of the journey to recovery is guided by our decreasing carelessness with cleaning and our increasing desire for biological youth.

---

178   Cogen AL, Nizet V, Gallo RL. **Skin microbiota: a source of disease or defence?** Br J Dermatol. 2008 Mar;158(3):442-55. *pubmed.gov/18275522*

179   Piérard-Franchimont C, Xhauflaire-Uhoda E, Piérard GE. **Revisiting dandruff.** Int J Cosmet Sci. 2006 Oct;28(5):311-8. *pubmed.gov/18489295*

180   Wikipedia. **Oral microbiology.** Accessed 2016. *en.wikipedia.org/wiki/Oral_microbiology*

181   Yu YH, Chasman DI, Buring JE, Rose L, Ridker PM. **Cardiovascular risks associated with incident and prevalent periodontal disease.** J Clin Periodontol. 2015 Jan;42(1):21-8. *pubmed.gov/25385537*

182   Noble JM, Scarmeas N, Celenti RS, Elkind MS, Wright CB, Schupf N, Papapanou PN. **Serum IgG antibody levels to periodontal microbiota are associated with incident Alzheimer disease.** PLoS One. 2014 Dec 18;9(12):e114959. *pubmed.gov/25522313*

While TR Skincare targets skin and hair directly, the other recovery behaviors nourish them from the inside. The link between inner health and outward health is highlighted in the following research studies.

Metabolic fitness and facial aging. TR Strength and Sustenance increase metabolic fitness. The Duke University study on biological age discussed in *Chapter Two: Metabolic Fitness* shows that people with higher metabolic fitness have slower facial aging.[**Duke Study**]

Obesity and hair loss. TR Strength and Sustenance reduce obesity. Obesity can increase the risk of male-pattern baldness up to 250% and early-onset male-pattern baldness up to 400%.[**183**]

Metabolic syndrome and hair loss. TR Strength and Sustenance reduce the risk of metabolic syndrome. Early-onset male-pattern baldness can associate with a 175% increased prevalence of metabolic syndrome.[**184**]

Blood sugar and perceived age. TR Strength and Sustenance reduce blood sugar levels. Lower blood sugar is associated with a lower perceived age.[**185**]

Dietary carotenoids and perceived health. TR Sustenance increases dietary carotenoids from fruits and vegetables which causes a subtle but perceptible change in facial skin color. Facial skin carotenoids raise perceived healthiness AND physical attractiveness.[**186**] Facial skin carotenoids are even perceived as more

183 Yang CC, Hsieh FN, Lin LY, Hsu CK, Sheu HM, Chen W. **Higher body mass index is associated with greater severity of alopecia in men with male-pattern androgenetic alopecia in Taiwan: a cross-sectional study.** J Am Acad Dermatol. 2014 Feb;70(2):297-302.e1. *pubmed. gov/24184140*

184 Banger HS, Malhotra SK, Singh S, Mahajan M. **Is Early Onset Androgenic Alopecia a Marker of Metabolic Syndrome and Carotid Artery Atherosclerosis in Young Indian Male Patients?** Int J Trichology. 2015 Oct-Dec;7(4):141-7. *pubmed.gov/26903742*

185 Noordam R, Gunn DA, Tomlin CC, Maier AB, Mooijaart SP, Slagboom PE, Westendorp RG, de Craen AJ, van Heemst D; Leiden Longevity Study Group. **High serum glucose levels are associated with a higher perceived age.** Age (Dordr). 2013 Feb;35(1):189-95. *pubmed.gov/22102339*

186 Whitehead RD, Re D, Xiao D, Ozakinci G, Perrett DI. **You are what**

healthy AND more attractive than a suntan.[187]

Blood sugar, stress, and growth hormones. TR Strength simultaneously reduces blood sugar levels, reduces cortisol levels and increases growth hormone levels.[188] All these effects contribute to a lower perceived age.[189]

Skin fat content and perceived age. TR Strength and Sustenance reduce skin fat content. TR Skincare reduces photodamage. Both increased skin fat content and photodamage contribute to perceived facial age.[190]

Perceived age and survival. While all three parts of recovery lifestyle lower perceived age, there is an even bigger benefit — survival. Lower perceived age reduces the incidence of death in older age groups by up to 30%.[191]

RECOVERY LIFESTYLE AND THE FIVE FITNESSES

It should now be evident that the recovery behaviors in the recovery

you eat: within-subject increases in fruit and vegetable consumption confer beneficial skin-color changes. PLoS One. 2012;7(3):e32988. *pubmed.gov/22412966*

187 Lefevre CE, Perrett DI. **Fruit over sunbed: carotenoid skin colouration is found more attractive than melanin colouration.** Q J Exp Psychol (Hove). 2015;68(2):284-93. *pubmed.gov/25014019*

188 Sheikholeslami-Vatani D, Ahmadi S, Salavati R. **Comparison of the Effects of Resistance Exercise Orders on Number of Repetitions, Serum IGF-1, Testosterone and Cortisol Levels in Normal-Weight and Obese Men.** Asian J Sports Med. 2016 Mar 1;7(1):e30503. *pubmed.gov/27217934*

189 van Drielen K, Gunn DA, Noordam R, Griffiths CE, Westendorp RG, de Craen AJ, van Heemst D. **Disentangling the effects of circulating IGF-1, glucose, and cortisol on features of perceived age.** Age (Dordr). 2015 Jun;37(3):9771. *pubmed.gov/25874752*

190 Henderson AJ, Holzleitner IJ, Talamas SN, Perrett DI. **Perception of health from facial cues.** Philos Trans R Soc Lond B Biol Sci. 2016 May 5;371(1693). pii: 20150380. *pubmed.gov/27069057*

191 Uotinen V, Rantanen T, Suutama T. **Perceived age as a predictor of old age mortality: a 13-year prospective study.** Age Ageing. 2005 Jul; 34(4):368-72. *pubmed.gov/15899910*

lifestyle — considered individually — should not seem wildly OUT-LANDISH. But when we put them all together, they may seem wildly AMBITIOUS.

The recovery behaviors work together to strengthen the five fitnesses as follows:

	Five fitnesses				
TR Strength	*Met.*	*Circ.*	*Micr.*	*Imm.*	*Ment.*
Train like a hunter	✓	✓	✓	✓	✓
Sleep like a hunter	✓	✓	✓	✓	✓
TR Sustenance	*Met.*	*Circ.*	*Micr.*	*Imm.*	*Ment.*
Eat like a gatherer	✓		✓	✓	✓
Cook like a gatherer	✓			✓	✓
Rest like a gatherer	✓	✓			✓
TR Skincare	*Met.*	*Circ.*	*Micr.*	*Imm.*	*Ment.*
Suit-up like a cosmonaut	✓		✓	✓	
Prepare like a cosmonaut	✓		✓	✓	

TR is mostly a head game. It's all about using humor to put some distance between us and all the zombie behaviors in the Western lifestyle. And, it's about forming crisp, positive images of recovery behaviors to make the journey more rewarding. TR is designed to make the Western lifestyle less seductive and the C word more satisfying.[192]

THE ESCALATOR OF AGE

TR proposes a metaphor called the Escalator of Age to describe what happens to us when we are infected with zombie viruses and we take our fitness for granted. Like any escalator, the Escalator of Age takes no effort on our part and carries us forward in age while we relax and enjoy ourselves. It carries us forward while we neglect our fitness. It carries us forward while we wait for someone else to fix our frailty.

The recovery lifestyle shows us how to counter the downward flow of the Escalator of Age. The recovery lifestyle allows us to match our walking speed to the speed of a treadmill, so we remain stationary while the conveyer belt moves below us. The recovery lifestyle turns the Escalator of Age into a Treadmill of Youth.

---

192 Wikipedia. **Conscientiousness.** Accessed 2016. *en.wikipedia.org/wiki/Conscientiousness*

As we begin adopting the recovery lifestyle and begin preserving youthfulness and fitness, we'll notice differences between ourselves and our fellow zombies. We'll become aware of the Escalator of Age carrying our fellow zombies. We'll find our footing and rhythm on the Treadmill of Youth.

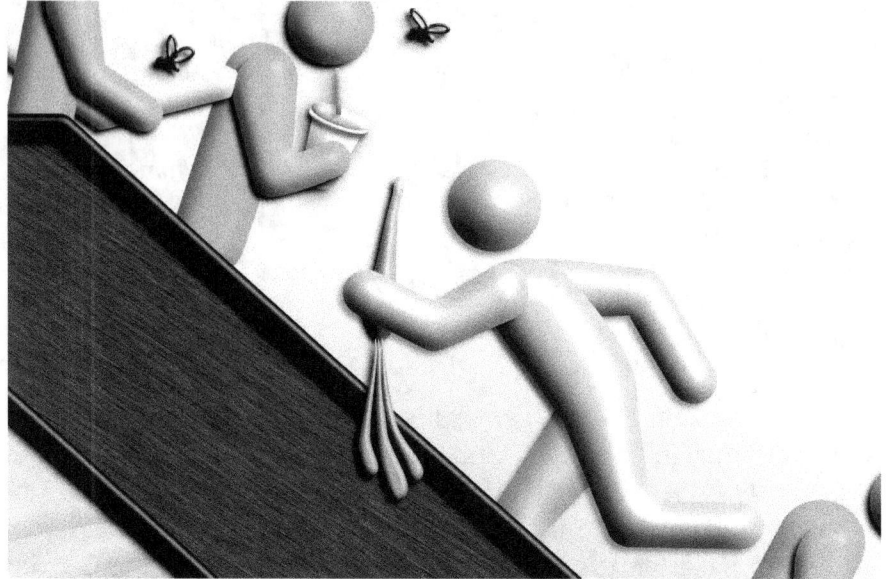

Using the Escalator of Age as a Treadmill of Youth.

We'll also become more aware of the full-throttle zombies in our lives. We'll notice they're not standing patiently on the Escalator. They're walking down the escalator. They encourage zombies to come along with them, so they require more finesse to dodge.

Surprisingly, we may begin to enjoy watching the other zombies on the Escalator. In particular, when full-throttle zombies indulge in zombie food, we can vicariously SAVOR their enjoyment. We'll be surprised how motivating Total Recovery becomes when we transition from people watching to zombie watching.

So, on behalf of all zombies in recovery, we should express our gratitude to the full-throttle zombies in our lives. Keep doing what you're doing. You're really helping us out. Perhaps we can return the favor. Have the next one on us. Just tell us which flavor and how much. Cheers!

The Treadmill of Youth is supported by all the research presented in the previous chapters. It's supported by research studies on the C word. Most of all, it's supported by research studies on people using ACTUAL treadmills.

Cardiac patients on a treadmill. Italian researchers confirm an ACTUAL treadmill can predict longevity. They measure the average walking speed of over 1200 cardiac patients ages 25 to 85. When they monitor the patients over eight years, they observe the faster walking patients have an increased rate of survival — by up to 80%. [**193**]

Adults on a treadmill. Johns Hopkins researchers confirm the treadmill test works with healthy adults too. They assess the treadmill fitness of 58,000 adults ages 18 to 96 who are free of heart disease and then follow them for 10 years. They observe that the adults with greater treadmill fitness are more likely to survive over the 10-year period of follow-up.[**194**]

Older adults on a treadmill. University of Pittsburgh researchers confirm walking speed alone can predict survival in older adults. The researchers pool the data from nine studies spanning over 34,000 individuals ages 65 and older. They confirm that walking speed predicts survival better than existing chronic conditions, smoking history, blood pressure, body mass index, and hospitalization status.[**195**]

---

193   Chiaranda G, Bernardi E, Codecà L, Conconi F, Myers J, Terranova F, Volpato S, Mazzoni G, Grazzi G. **Treadmill walking speed and survival prediction in men with cardiovascular disease: a 10-year follow-up study.** BMJ Open. 2013 Oct 25;3(10):e003446. *pubmed.gov/ 24163203*

194   Ahmed HM, Al-Mallah MH, McEvoy JW, Nasir K, Blumenthal RS, Jones SR, Brawner CA, Keteyian SJ, Blaha MJ. **Maximal Exercise Testing Variables and 10-Year Survival: Fitness Risk Score Derivation From the FIT Project.** Mayo Clin Proc. 2015 Mar;90(3):346-55. *pubmed.gov/25744114*

195   Studenski S, Perera S, Patel K, Rosano C, Faulkner K, Inzitari M, Brach J, Chandler J, Cawthon P, Connor EB, Nevitt M, Visser M, Kritchevsky S, Badinelli S, Harris T, Newman AB, Cauley J, Ferrucci L, Guralnik J. **Gait speed and survival in older adults.** JAMA. 2011 Jan 5;305(1):50-8. *pubmed.gov/21205966*

The Treadmill of Youth is real. Researchers see evidence of it whenever they study fitness and youthfulness. TR is real. TR incorporates fitness, nutrition, and skincare to keep us on the Treadmill of Youth as long as possible — as naturally as possible.

ZOMBIE YEARS

We'll now discuss how lifestyle influences the rate of biological aging and how to represent the rate as zombie years. Let's start by considering how the following full-throttle zombie behaviors speed up aging.

- *Sun tanning* accelerates aging of skin.[196]
- *Smoking* accelerates aging of the lungs and skin.[197]
- *Obesity* accelerates aging of internal organs and skin.[198]
- *Chronic stress* accelerates aging of internal organs and skin. [199]

We should expect zombie viruses to continue mutating and continue promoting new zombie behaviors that accelerate biological aging.

We discussed how lifestyle stress contributes to aging in *Chapter Four: Biological Age*. The rate of biological aging is represented by the lifestyle coefficient (C_L). This term is rather technical and is really meant for fellow scientists and health professionals. The term may not catch on with the general public.

But in the near future, the general public will start to notice the differences in aging between full-throttle zombies and zombies in recovery. Even full-throttle zombies will notice that something's up. We'll need some way to describe it.

Say hello to ZOMBIE YEARS.

They're like dog years, but they're different for each type of

196 Wikipedia. **Photoaging.** Accessed 2016. *en.wikipedia.org/wiki/Photoaging*

197 Wikipedia. **Health effects of tobacco.** Accessed 2016. *en.wikipedia.org/wiki/Health_effects_of_tobacco*

198 Wikipedia. **Obesity-associated morbidity.** Accessed 2016. *en.wikipedia.org/wiki/Obesity-associated_morbidity*

199 Wikipedia. **Chronic stress.** Accessed 2016. *en.wikipedia.org/wiki/Chronic_stress*

zombie. They're depicted below in the *Zombie Years Plot*. They help us compute our biological age from our calendar age for each type of zombie behavior.

ZOMBIE YEARS PLOT

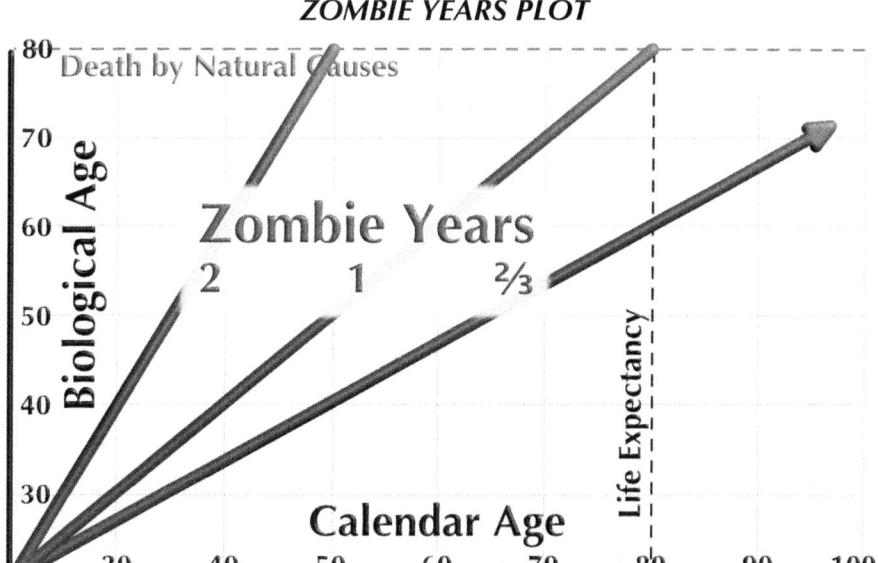

Normal zombie. A normal zombie RELAXES on the Escalator of Age, causing them to age ONE zombie year every calendar year. They go from biological age 20 to 80 in the typical 60 calendar years. They have a lifespan of 80 calendar years, consistent with the average U.S. adult.

Full-throttle zombie. A full-throttle zombie WALKS DOWN the Escalator of Age, causing them to age TWO zombie years every calendar year. They go from biological age 20 to 80 in only 30 calendar years. They have a lifespan of 50 calendar years, consistent with the fastest aging U.S. adults.

Recovering zombie. A recovering zombie WALKS AGAINST the Escalator of Age, causing them to age TWO-THIRDS of a zombie year every calendar year. They go from biological age 20 to 80 in a whopping 90 calendar years. They have a lifespan of 110 calendar years, consistent with the slowest of the slow aging U.S. adults.

Currently, 1 in 10 U.S. adults who survive past age 20 have a lifespan of 97 calendar years, which means they age 0.77 zombie years every calendar year. Only about 1 in 100,000 U.S. adults live to age 110, which means they age $^2/_3$ zombie years per calendar year.

We need more people walking against the Escalator of Age. It's good to be optimistic, especially now that we have Total Recovery.

The *Zombie Years Plot* should look similar to the *Lifestyle Coefficient Plot* presented in *Chapter Four: Biological Age*. That's because they're nearly identical. Just the names have been changed to protect the innocent. The plot should also look like the *Hayflick Coefficient Plot* presented in *Chapter Four*.

All three plots pretty much represent the same thing but at different levels of technical detail. The Hayflick coefficient (C_H) is for laboratory researchers. The lifestyle coefficient (C_L) is for clinical researchers. And zombie years are for the rest of us.

DOG YEARS REVISITED

Zombie years even help us to understand dog years. Dog years are different for a small dog and a giant dog. A small dog typically lives 16 years. A giant dog typically lives only 8 years. A medium dog lives somewhere between 10 to 13 years.[**200**]

Aging rates. If we use biological age 80 as the life expectancy of a dog, then a small dog ages 5 dog years per calendar year, a medium dog ages 7 dog years per calendar year, and a giant dog ages 10 dog years per calendar year.

Exercise. A small dog gets more exercise than a giant dog because the small dog gets sufficient exercise space indoors or in a small yard. A small dog takes more steps than a big dog on a walk around the block.

Growth hormones. A small dog has fewer growth hormones circulating in its body compared to a giant dog. The growth hormones stress the cells in the giant dog and age it faster. (and yes, tall people suffer the same growth hormone stress.)

Age-related disorders. Dogs develop the same age-related features as people: reduced activity, weight gain, diabetes, cancer, and senility. They also suffer loss of teeth, muscle, bone, vision, hearing, bladder control, skin elasticity, hair, and hair color.

---

200 Wikipedia. **Aging in dogs.** Accessed 2016. *en.wikipedia.org/wiki/Aging_in_dogs*

Giant dogs. Being a giant dog is hard on the dog body in a similar way that being a full-throttle zombie is hard on the human body.

Small dogs. Being a small dog is gentle on the dog body in a similar way that being a recovering zombie is gentle on the human body.

THE BENEFIT OF ZOMBIE YEARS

We know how dog owners enjoy using dog years to estimate the biological age of their dogs.

Zombies will enjoy zombie years for the same reason. In particular, full-throttle zombies have such compressed lifespans they'll need to make every moment count. They could even use their age in zombie years to get special treatment and cut in line.

- *At restaurants* — "In zombie years, I qualify for the tuesday special."
- *While shopping* — " In zombie years, I qualify for the motorized cart and the free assistance back to my car."
- *Airport security* — " In zombie years, I qualify for the short line on the side."
- *Airplane boarding* — " In zombie years, I qualify for pre-boarding."

Full-throttle zombies will want to buy high-tech mobility devices to zoom around in. High-tech gadget stores will start selling mobility devices to them. Toy stores will start selling mobility devices just for the little zombies.

Full-throttle zombies will demand more services accessible from their mobility devices. Restaurants could build custom drive-up windows, custom entrances, check-out lanes, passing lanes, pit-stop crews, and charging stations.

Full-throttle zombies will want to buy bigger trucks for driving on the road. They'll want louder horns to intimidate the rest of us to get out of their way. They'll make every lane the fast lane as they sprint head-long toward the finish line.

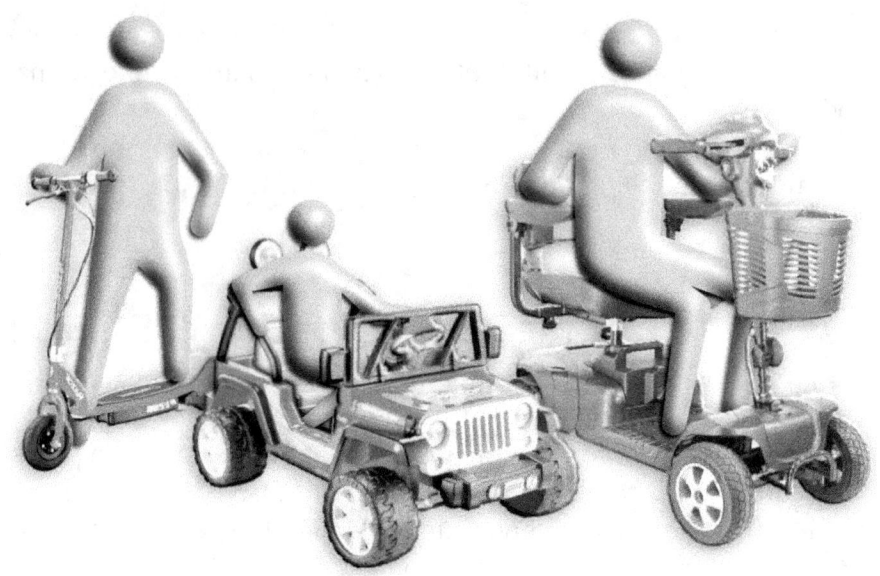

High-tech mobility devices.

The clock is ticking fast for full-throttle zombies. It's about time we yield them more space to pass.

THE CLASH OF THE ZOMBIES

Full-throttle zombies and recovering zombies may grow increasingly apart in lifestyle and in culture. These differences may lead to clashes. Instead of letting things get out of hand, consider how these clashes can be resolved with zombie years.

Full-throttle zombies often park in handicapped spots so they can hurry up. They often display handicapped placards on their cars even though they hop out with two working feet and two working legs. They walk so fast, we can't catch up with them to ask why they need to park in handicapped. Inside each of us is a voice that screams,

> *"Maybe if you parked farther away and walked a little more, you wouldn't need the handicapped placard."*

Zombie years help us all understand their need for speed. Zombie years might encourage merchants to set aside more dual-use parking spots for handicapped and for full-throttle zombies. Zombies wouldn't need to fake being handicapped, and the rest of us would back off. We'd stop arguing with full-throttle zombies about parking in handicapped. We'd start appreciating the differences in our zombie years as we walk the longer distances from our remote parking spaces.

Consider how full-throttle zombies drive enormous diesel-guzzling vehicles. On occasion, they disable their emission systems to make thick smoke. They call it ROLLING COAL.[201] They spew diesel soot at pedestrians, bicyclists, and drivers of fuel-efficient cars. They film themselves rolling coal, and they post it online. Full-throttle zombies find this kind of behavior absolutely hilarious. They proudly proclaim that air pollution is irrelevant, climate change is fake, and environmentalism is a joke.

Zombie years help us all understand their unique point of view. We would all agree that climate change is negligible within such short zombie years. Full-throttle zombies don't prioritize their own health, so why should they prioritize the health of the environment? Taking care of the environment is for people with more time on their hands.

Zombie years might encourage merchants to offer in-home services to help keep full-throttle zombies off the road, out of their parking lots, and somewhere safe to live their fast and voracious lives. Merchants might offer them enhanced cable subscriptions with bonus sports channels, along with pizza, soda, and cigarette delivery — anything to keep our roads more safe, to keep our air more fresh, and to speed up every zombie year clock.

Zombie years would help us stop arguing with each other about air pollution and climate change. Full-throttle zombies would enjoy their shorter years with better in-home services, and the rest of us would enjoy our longer years with safer roads and fresher air.

---

201 Wikipedia. **Rolling coal.** Accessed 2016. *en.wikipedia.org/wiki/Rolling_coal*

CHAPTER SEVEN REVIEW

TR Strength

Train like a hunter includes daily strength training, endurance training, and stretching. These recovery behaviors strengthen metabolic and mental fitness.

Sleep like a hunter includes going to bed at the same time every night, sleeping seven hours every night, getting up at the same time every morning, and avoiding long naps every day. These recovery behaviors strengthen all five fitnesses.

TR Sustenance

Eat like a gatherer means categorizing foods according to whether they are nourishing or snacks. Nourishing foods are the subset of foods that the Paleolithic and Vegetarian diets come closest to agreement on. They include fruits, vegetables, beans, and nuts as the staple foods. Snack foods include meat, dairy, wheat, rice, and processed foods. Eating more nourishing foods and less snack foods strengthens metabolic, microbial, immune, and mental fitness.

Cook like a gatherer means preparing nourishing foods raw or by steaming, stewing, or microwaving them. COOK LIKE A HUNTER means preparing foods by roasting, frying, grilling, and smoking them which causes ANY food to become a snack food. Cooking like a gatherer strengthens metabolic fitness (by reducing food carcinogenicity) and immune fitness (by reducing food inflammation).

Rest like a gatherer means eating during the daytime and fasting during the evening and night. It reduces nutrient stress and increases cellular recycling and repair. It strengthens all five fitnesses.

TR Skincare

Suit-up like a cosmonaut means regularly applying sunscreen to reduce ultraviolet radiation stress, applying moisturizer to reduce dehydration stress, applying topical anti-oxidants to reduce oxidation stress, and applying essential oils to support skin microbial balance and reduce inflammation stress. These recovery behaviors strengthen the metabolic, microbial, and immune fitness of the skin and hair follicles.

Prepare like a cosmonaut means regularly washing the face and body and regularly cleaning the teeth. These recovery behaviors strengthen the metabolic, microbial, and immune fitness of the skin, mouth, and surprisingly, the heart, brain, and other internal organs.

Escalator of age. This metaphor represents what happens when zombies are lulled into complacency by the quick-fix zombie virus. Normal zombies relax on the escalator and age gradually. Full-throttle zombies walk forward down the escalator and age faster.

Treadmill of youth. This metaphor represents what happens when the recovering zombie neutralizes the quick-fix zombie virus and takes responsibility for the fitness of their body. The recovering zombie strengthens the five fitnesses and jogs backwards against the flow of the Escalator as if it were a treadmill.

Zombie years. This term describes the speed of biological aging caused by lifestyle. Zombie years are like dog years, but they're for humans, and they only apply to the period of adulthood starting at calendar age 20. Adulthood is when biological aging is most sensitive to the influence of lifestyle.

Biological age is defined to have an end point of 80, corresponding to death by natural causes. Calendar age, however, has an ambiguous end point because lifestyle determines how many calendar years are needed to reach death by natural causes.

For each type of zombie behavior, a person accumulates a different number of zombie years each calendar year until they reach biological age 80. A person could reach biological age 80 as early as calendar age 50 and as late as calendar age 110.

Zombie Behavior	Zombie Years	Calendar Age at Death
Full-throttle	2	50
Normal	1	80
Recovering	$^2/_3$	110

CHAPTER SEVEN IMAGINE

For fun, we can imagine what happens when we mix and match every recovery behavior with every archetypal figure. Notice how one pairing is ideal while the other possible pairings are less ideal and are somewhat humorous.

RECOVERY LIFESTYLE JUMBLE

TR Strength	Hunter	Gatherer	Cosmonaut
Train like a ...	✓	Weak muscles	No gravity
Sleep like a ...	✓	Sleep in fear	No day/night
TR Sustenance	**Hunter**	**Gatherer**	**Cosmonaut**
Eat like a ...	Too much meat	✓	Over-processed
Cook like a ...	Over-grilled	✓	Over-processed
Rest like a ...	Night feasting	✓	No day/night
TR Skincare	**Hunter**	**Gatherer**	**Cosmonaut**
Suit up like a ...	UV exposed	UV exposed	✓
Prepare like a ...	Under-washed	Under-washed	✓

Now let's imagine what the Western lifestyle would look like with its zombie behaviors matched with the same archetypal figures.

WESTERN LIFESTYLE JUMBLE

Zombie Strength	Hunter	Gatherer	Cosmonaut
Train like a ...		✓	?
Sleep like a ...		?	✓
Zombie Sustenance	**Hunter**	**Gatherer**	**Cosmonaut**
Eat like a ...	✓		✓
Cook like a ...	✓		✓
Rest like a ...	✓		✓
Zombie Skincare	**Hunter**	**Gatherer**	**Cosmonaut**
Suit up like a ...	✓	✓	
Prepare like a ...	✓	✓	

Race to the Finish

Consider how biological age has a clear END POINT. It is death by natural causes. But calendar age has no clear end point. Biological aging is clear-cut. Calendar aging is ambiguous.

The end point of biological age is like a finish line at the end of a race. The full-throttle zombie races to the finish line with astounding speed. The recovering zombie inches toward the finish line like a slow poke. Zombie years describe the speed at which each zombie moves toward the finish line.

The finish line and zombie years are reminiscent of the allegorical race between the tortoise and the hare. Let's imagine an updated version just for us zombies and our littlest zombies.

Let's imagine how upon reaching adulthood, the zombie rabbit challenges the zombie turtle to a race.

The zombie rabbit sprints to an early lead with a performance enhancing diet of hot dogs and Big Gulps. The zombie rabbit keeps sprinting and sprinting. It maintains a non-stop, break-neck, full-throttle zombie sprint to the finish line — of death by natural causes. With its giant soda cup, the zombie rabbit laughs, taunts, and shuffles across the finish line.

The zombie turtle shrugs it off. It looks around. It looks to see if there's another zombie rabbit who wants to race.

LIFESTYLE TRANSMITTED DISEASE

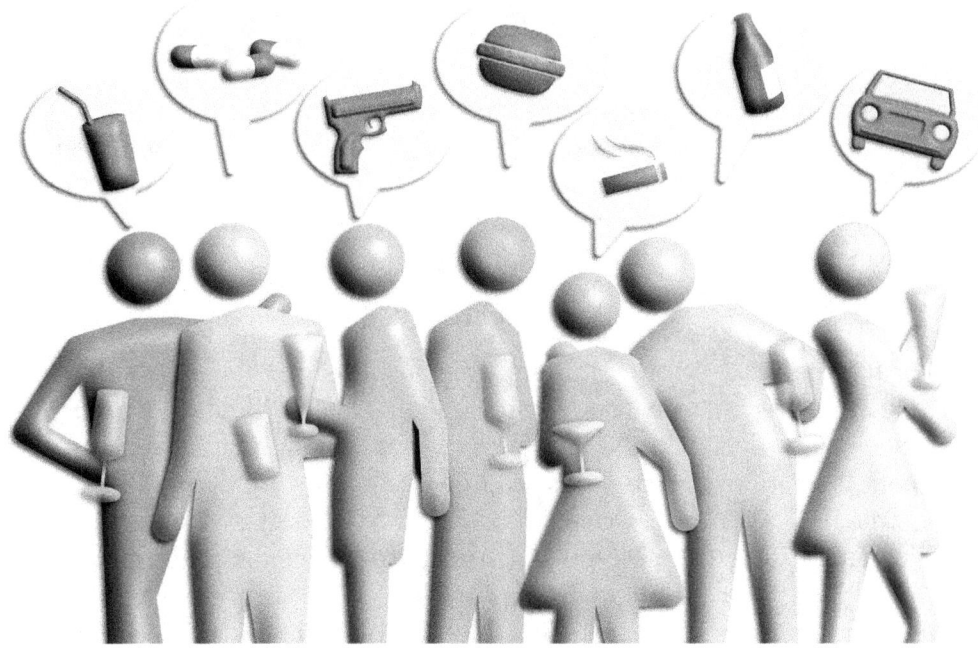

Social intercourse transmits lifestyle that transmits disease.

Our Western lifestyle leads us toward chronic disease. Health professionals know our lifestyle is the problem, yet they cannot get us to change. The more they tell us about healthy behaviors and unhealthy behaviors, the more exhausted we get and the less we do about it. We need to consider how the concept of lifestyle transmitted disease can help us.

In this chapter, we examine the following topics:
- *Remember NCDs?*
- *LTDs and STDs.*
- *The LTD yuck factor.*
- *Learning from our mistakes.*
- *The Western lifestyle goes viral.*
- *Restaurants transmit LTDs.*

- *Family and friends transmit LTDs.*
- *The LTD concept is prophylactic.*
- *LTDs lurking in plain sight.*
- *Review.*
- *Imagine.*

REMEMBER NCDs?

As discussed in *Chapter Five: Zombie Behaviors*, health professionals classify a disease caused by lifestyle or by exposure to pollution as a non-communicable disease (NCD). Non-communicable means the disease is not transmitted by a pathogen between people. NCDs are increasing as our lifestyles change and as our environmental pollution increases.[**202**]

The NCD concept is useful for particular researchers, but not for the rest of us. Non-communicable suggests no one is at fault. It does not help us see how we're inflicting these diseases on ourselves by our personal behaviors or by our polluting of the environment. And it does not help us see how we can avoid them. It lets us off the hook. It lets everyone off the hook. NCDs just … happen.

NCD is a troublesome term because it neglects the zombie viruses passed to us by advertisers and that we pass on to each other. Zombie viruses are highly infectious and communicable. Zombie viruses help explain how the NCD epidemic spreads. Zombie viruses are endemic to the Western lifestyle — a lifestyle recognized by its zombie behaviors more than its recovery behaviors. Zombie viruses spread from Western countries to developing countries, and they spread the epidemic of NCDs.

The United Nations and the World Health Organization are leading a global effort to prevent NCDs. Unfortunately, any effort based on cajoling us to live healthier will fail if it neglects the role of zombie viruses and zombie behaviors. You can lead a zombie to water, but you can't make them exercise in it.

In Total Recovery, we use terms such as zombie behaviors, zombie viruses, and the journey to recovery to help combat NCDs. But health professionals may not be comfortable using these terms.

---

202 Wikipedia. **Non-communicable disease.** Accessed 2016. *en.wikipedia.org/wiki/Non-communicable_disease*

They need a term that is better suited for doctors' offices and research seminars. They need a term that encapsulates how LIFESTYLE is the MECHANISM for disease transmission.

Say hello to *lifestyle transmitted disease*.

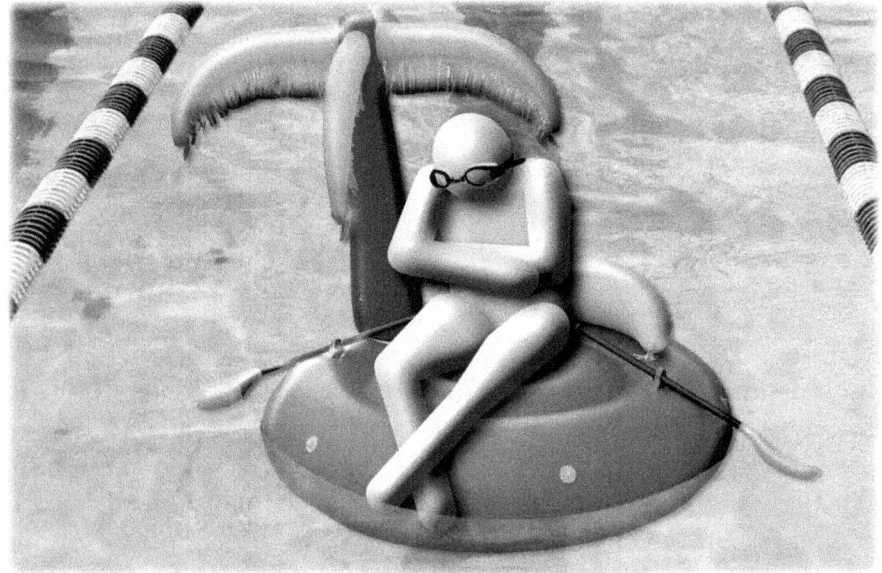

You can lead a zombie to water ...

LTDs AND STDs

TR proposes that we replace the troublesome concept of non-communicable disease with lifestyle transmitted disease (LTD) — which is based on the concept of sexually transmitted disease.

When we adopt high-risk sexual behaviors, over time, we contract STDs. Typical STDs are chlamydia, gonorrhea, herpes, and HIV.[203] When we adopt unhealthy or environmentally polluting behaviors, over time, we contract LTDs. Typical LTDs are lung disease, type 2 diabetes, cardiovascular disease, inflammatory bowel disease, fatty liver disease, and Alzheimer's disease.

LTD also represents DISORDER which is an unhealthy state leading to disease. Typical lifestyle transmitted DISORDERS include: asthma, obesity, high blood pressure, high blood sugar, high blood lipids, and irritable bowel syndrome. Traditionally, disorders

203 Wikipedia. **Sexually transmitted disease.** Accessed 2016. *en. wikipedia.org/wiki/Sexually_transmitted_disease*

become more common as adults age, but disorders are increasingly prevalent among adolescents. When we pass along unhealthy behaviors to our children or we pollute our environment, over time, our children contract LTDs.

NCDs are often called LIFESTYLE diseases. This term almost works, but it's awkward. If we have heart disease, our HEART may die, but when we have a lifestyle disease, our LIFESTYLE will not die.[204] We will die before our lifestyle will. Lifestyle is the TRANSMITTER of disease.

The LTD concept shines a spotlight on what we're doing to our bodies. These diseases don't just happen. They're self-inflicted by our zombie behaviors. The LTD concept puts the onus back on us as custodians of our bodies.

The LTD concept also shines a spotlight on what we're doing to the environment. Pollution of the air, soil, and water doesn't just happen. It's inflicted by our zombie behaviors.

Our exposure to the pollution causes disorder and disease in our bodies. These LTDs don't just happen. They are inflicted on us by the pollution caused by our zombie behaviors and the zombie products we buy.

The LTD concept puts the onus back on us as custodians of our clean air, our clean water, and our fragile planet.

To help encourage the health community to adopt the LTD concept, I'm officially dedicating it to the public domain.[205] Please use it, adapt it, and nurture it in any way that helps you and the public good.

THE LTD YUCK FACTOR

The STD and LTD concepts work because they have a built-in yuck factor. They should make us think of yucky things inside our bodies.

---

204 Although it's kinda funny to think of a lifestyle disease leading to its own demise. "It was a lifestyle that tried its hardest until the very end. May it rest in peace..."

205 "LTD," "lifestyle transmitted disorder," and "lifestyle transmitted disease" are hereby dedicated to the public domain. All copyright ownership rights to these three concepts are waived under the Creative Commons Zero public domain dedication at *creativecommons.org/ publicdomain/zero/1.0*. Please help spread the word!

They should make us think of organs that are red, swollen, inflamed, pus-filled, and necrotic.

STDs make us think of inflamed mouths and genitals. LTDs should make us think of inflamed livers, pancreases, hearts, kidneys, and brains. When we routinely engage in zombie behaviors, over time, we cause our organs to become inflamed, which should seem yucky.

The STD and LTD concepts also work because they make us think twice about how we interact with each other. STDs are transmitted by SEXUAL intercourse.LTDs are transmitted by SOCIAL intercourse. Our zombie behaviors cause the transmission of yucky things.

LEARNING FROM OUR MISTAKES

LTDs should begin to sound like avoidable diseases. They should encourage us to think twice about our zombie behaviors. And when we contract LTDs, they'll help us own up to our zombie behaviors — just like when we contract STDs.

Imagine telling your friends,

> *"My doctor recommends I start eating healthy food because I keep getting LTDs."*

It should start to sound like you're saying,

> *"My doctor recommends I start using condoms because I keep getting STDs."*

These two concepts help us identify our zombie behaviors and replace them with recovery behaviors. Recovery behaviors and disease prevention are much better than zombie behaviors and chronic medication.

Are you starting to see how effective the LTD term is? And how much better it is than the NCD term? Do you even remember what NCD stands for? It's not easy. It's so boring it hurts. LTD is way better and way yuckier. It should help us think harder about our zombie behaviors and about what we can do differently.

THE WESTERN LIFESTYLE GOES VIRAL

Our Western lifestyle is transmitted from parent to child and from friend to friend. It's transmitted by food, beverage, tobacco, and alcohol companies. It's transmitted by film and broadcasting companies.

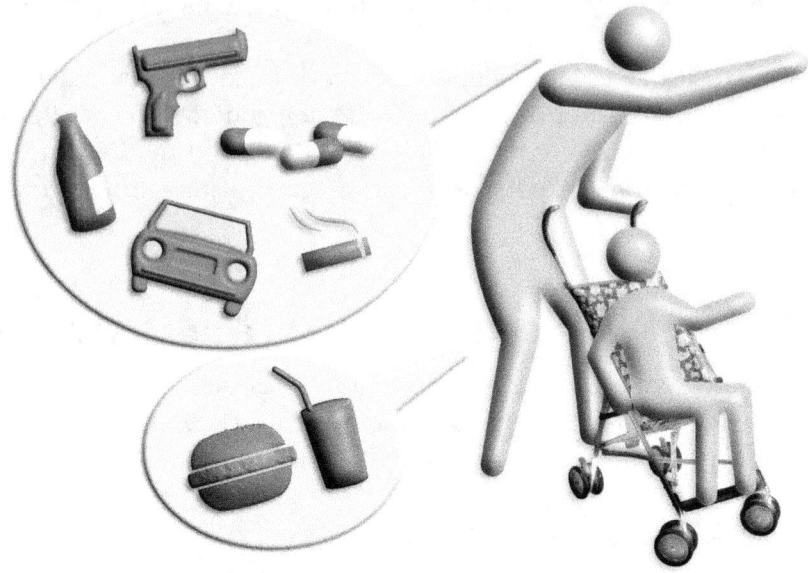

Lifestyle is transmitted from parent to child.

Our Western lifestyle is going viral. It's transmitted from rich countries to developing countries. Developing countries are facing LTD epidemics like ours. Worldwide deaths from LTDs keep climbing. Currently 68% of deaths are caused by LTDs.[**206**] Since lifestyle is an infectious agent, NON-COMMUNICABLE doesn't make sense. NCD is really a nonsense term because NCDs are 100% communicable.

The LTD concept highlights how our Western lifestyle is a pathogen and how each of us is a carrier.[**207**] The Western lifestyle infects our minds as a collection of zombie viruses which induces a repertoire of zombie behaviors.

The Western lifestyle provides us short-term pleasure, but it in-

---

206 Wikipedia. **Non-communicable disease.** Accessed 2016. *en.wikipedia.org/wiki/Non-communicable_disease*

207 Wikipedia. **Vector (epidemiology).** Accessed 2016. *en.wikipedia.org/wiki/Vector_(epidemiology)*

creases our long-term burden of LTDs. It provides corporations short-term profits, but it increases their long-term burden of employee health insurance.

Our lifestyle is causing an LTD epidemic here at home. It is causing an LTD pandemic across the globe.

Our healthcare community would benefit from the LTD term. They've been struggling to get people's attention about NCDs, but they've been hamstrung by the NCD term itself.

They may be concerned LTD is too provocative. But in the context of a public-awareness campaign, a provocative term is a good thing — a really good thing. Remember the "This is your brain on drugs" campaign with the eggs in the frypan? Remember the anti-smoking campaign with cigarette smoke coming out of people's tracheostomy holes?

Provocative is what GETS our attention. And humor is what KEEPS our attention.

RESTAURANTS TRANSMIT LTDs

The LTD yuck factor helps us resist the zombie viruses marketed to us. It's like how the STD yuck factor helps us resist the overt sexualization in our culture. It's a war of concepts, and it's time we have a fair fight.

We should feel inspired to walk into any fast food restaurant and demand they stop infecting us with LTDs. The employees will look confused next to their deep fryers and milk shake machines. They'll say they really don't know anything about LTDs.

Restaurants prevent food-borne infections by keeping their facilities shiny and squeaky clean. But, they still transmit LTDs in these squeaky clean facilities. The shiny facade likely misleads patrons about the risks.

Restaurants generally hire young and attractive employees, which may also mislead patrons. Young employees frequently contract the LTDs, and yet they remain asymptomatic because the incubation time for LTDs is typically longer than the length of their employment. Employees often move on to other jobs before manifesting LTD symptoms.

Patrons should not assess the LTD risk of a restaurant by its shiny facilities and young employees. They should assess it by the

LTD symptoms of other restaurant patrons. It's just like assessing the STD risk of a partner by the STD symptoms of former partners. Fellow restaurant patrons may already show full-blown LTD symptoms.

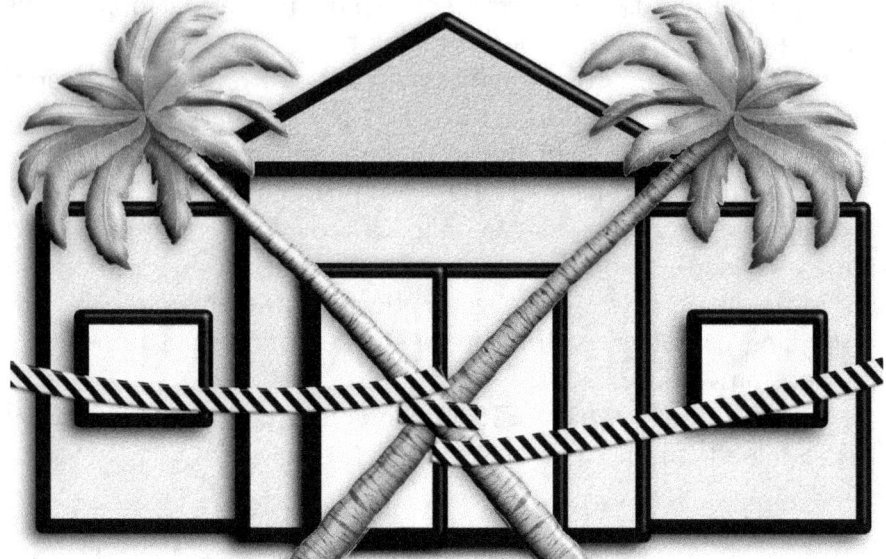

The shiny facade misleads patrons about the risks.

Many state laws require STD-infected individuals to inform their partners before they go to bed. We should require LTD-infected restaurants to inform their customers before they go IN-N-OUT.

FAMILY AND FRIENDS TRANSMIT LTDs

Family and friends also coerce us to eat LTD-transmitting foods. They love their food and they want us to love it too. But we must be vigilant when we share meals with anyone, whether it's a friend or a family member. It's just like being vigilant about sharing sex with an STD-infected partner.

The two scenarios are surprisingly similar and surprisingly awkward. Discussing LTDs and safe foods with a meal partner is as awkward as discussing STDs and safe sex with a sexual partner. In both cases, we don't want to hurt their feelings, and we don't want to ruin the mood. Both situations are awkward because they're both the same dilemma.

We can use the lessons learned in the control of STDs to guide how we control LTDs. Talking openly about STD testing and safe sex is analogous to talking openly about LTD testing and safe foods. It's the same awkwardness that requires the same level of openness and honesty to resolve.

To demonstrate the equivalence of these two scenarios, we'll examine STD health advice given by the U.S. government.[208] Their health pamphlet is called STD Testing: Conversation Starters. But, we'll substitute the following STD terms with LTD terms:

- Substitute STD with LTD,
- Substitute HAVE SEX with SHARE FOOD, and
- Substitute USE CONDOMS with EAT GREENS.

Our new health pamphlet is called LTD TESTING: CONVERSATION STARTERS. The results are surprisingly relevant and fascinating.

LTD TESTING:
CONVERSATION STARTERS

It might be hard to talk to your partner about getting tested for LIFESTYLE TRANSMITTED DISEASES (LTDs), but it's important. Chances are your partner will be glad you brought it up.

TALK BEFORE you SHARE FOOD.

"Why take a chance when we can know for sure?"

"I was tested for LTDs. Are you willing to do the same?"

SHARE the FACTS.

"Many people who have an LTD don't know it."

"The sooner most LTDs are found, the easier they are to treat."

"Getting tested is easier than ever before. You may not even have to give blood."

---

208 Healthfinder.gov. **STD Testing: Conversation starters.** Office of Disease Prevention and Health Promotion. U.S. Department of Health and Human Services. Accessed 2016. *healthfinder.gov/HealthTopics/ Category/health-conditions-and-diseases/hiv-and-other-stds/std-testing-conversation-starters*

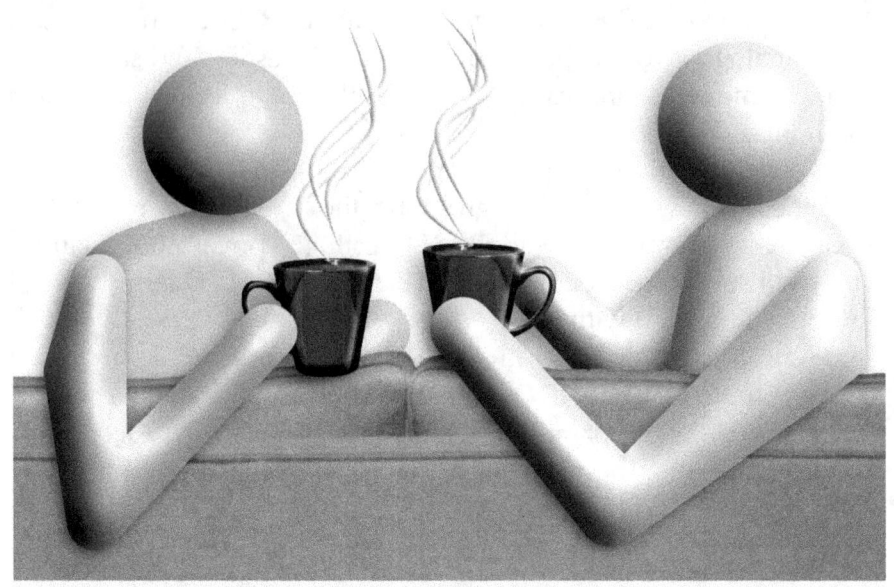

SHOW *THAT* **YOU CARE.**

"I really care about you. I want to make sure we are both healthy."

"Let's get tested together."

AGREE TO STAY SAFE.

"If we're going to SHARE FOOD, EATING GREENS is the best way to protect us from LTDs."

"Let's EAT GREENS every time we SHARE FOOD."

"We can enjoy SHARING FOOD more if we know it's safe."

THE **LTD CONCEPT** IS **PROPHYLACTIC**

Just bringing up the LTD concept in conversation tends to cool people's urges. It's like bringing up the STD concept. They both help people cool down and think clearly. The LTD concept has power all by itself. It's a prophylactic that encourages us and our meal partners to make healthy food choices — that are consistent with our overall lifestyle goals.

Here are some examples of how we may use the LTD concept

as a prophylactic in our conversations.

If our friend encourages us to "live a little" and try their double-double-cheeseburger, we might say,

"Did you hear you can get LTDs from it?"

We might continue,

"I don't know how often you put it in your mouth, but you might wanna get yourself tested for LTDs. And if you share it with your partner, your partner should get tested too."

This kind of conversation can help people control their urges and think more clearly. Our meal partner might even stop chewing. They might even lose their appetite for their LTD-infested double-double-cheeseburger and leave the rest on their plate.

They may be disappointed we're not sharing food with them. But they'll get over it. They'll appreciate how we're asking to share food in a healthy way that's good for the long term relationship.

If grandma spoils our kids with snacks, we might say something like,

"I'm concerned you're passing your LTDs on to your grandchildren."

Grandma may be shocked. She may take it badly. But if she can work through her feelings, she may appreciate how we're asking to share food in a healthy way that's good for everyone.

This conversation may even get the attention of our kids. Out of earshot, they'll ask,

"Does grandma have LTDs?"

"Your grandmother made a lot of choices when she was younger. She probably wishes she could have a do-over."

Our kids may begin to see how the decisions they make now will affect them the rest of their lives. They may be grateful their parents and grandparents could talk so openly and honestly with each other. They may learn how to talk openly and honestly with their friends about LTDs and healthy foods.

Try to incorporate the LTD concept into your own decision-making and into conversations with friends and loved ones.

LTDs LURKING in PLAIN SIGHT

It's pretty humorous how STD conversations can translate directly into LTD conversations, nearly word for word. It gives us permission to talk about LTDs in a way that's rich in double-entendre. If you enjoy double-entendre, then it's a riot.

But it's also pretty startling. It's startling that nobody's noticed LTDs before. Nobody's noticed the connection between STDs and LTDs.

What have all of us zombies been thinking about all these years? Food and sexuality. Why haven't we made this connection before?

Artists and musicians make references to food and sexuality all the time.[209] We use food metaphors to describe people's sexual body parts all the time. People find great pleasure in combining food desires with sexual desires.[210]

It's startling that no one has yet connected the way sexual diseases are transmitted with the way diet and lifestyle diseases are transmitted. No one has yet proposed the concept diet or lifestyle transmitted disease. For some reason, when we start thinking about disease, we get all clinical and technical. Our imagination evaporates. Our creativity vanishes. And, most importantly, our sense of personal responsibility for our chronic diseases vanishes.

Somehow our minds struggle to think clinically AND imaginatively. Our Western culture has trained our minds not to mix the two. TR is going to change all that.

TR is like a hot scorching wind that will burn away all the nonsense boundaries we've set up in our minds. TR makes us think technically and imaginatively at the same time. It's going to expand our minds. You're going to love it.

---

209 Wikipedia. **Food and sexuality.** Accessed 2016. *en.wikipedia.org/wiki/Food_and_sexuality*

210 Wikipedia. **Food play.** Accessed 2016. *en.wikipedia.org/wiki/Food_play*

CHAPTER EIGHT REVIEW

Non-communicable disease. This concept represents the diseases NOT transmitted by pathogens between people. This concept implies that diseases happen spontaneously without cause. This concept should be abandoned.

Lifestyle transmitted disorder and disease. This new concept represents disorders and diseases caused by our behaviors and by our environment. It's TRANSMITTED by a pathogen called LIFESTYLE. This concept highlights how disease has a clear mechanism of transmission. This concept should be used instead of non-communicable disease.

The Western lifestyle is a pathogenic lifestyle transmitted between people by social intercourse. The Western lifestyle pollutes the environment and causes climate change that in turn contributes to health disorder and disease.

Zombie viruses contribute to the transmission of the Western lifestyle. Zombie corporations spread them BETWEEN communities. Fellow zombies spread them WITHIN communities.

LTD prevention campaigns can adopt lessons learned from the STD prevention campaigns. LTD prevention efforts should try to discourage risky behaviors. LTD detection efforts should encourage testing when risky behaviors occur.

CHAPTER EIGHT IMAGINE

LTDs arise from risky zombie behaviors which are addressed by the recovery behaviors as follows:

ZOMBIE Behaviors	RECOVERY Behaviors
Zombie Strength	TR Strength
Sedentary behaviors	Train like a hunter
Poor sleep behaviors	Sleep like a hunter
Zombie Sustenance	TR Sustenance
Eating processed foods	Eat like a gatherer
Eating grilled foods	Cook like a gatherer
Eating late in the evening	Rest like a gatherer
Zombie Skincare	TR Skincare
Overexposure to UV	Suit up like a cosmonaut
Over-/under-washing	Prepare like a cosmonaut

In every case, our behaviors can be carefree and risky, or

they can be sensible and safe. Our behaviors can either promote LTDs, or they can fight LTDs.

Once we consider how zombie behaviors are carefree and risky behaviors, we can see how sexual behaviors and drug use behaviors fit into the concept of LTDs. Because sexual behavior is a lifestyle behavior, then an STD must also be an LTD. And because injection drug use behavior is another lifestyle behavior, then any STD contracted from injection drug use must also be an LTD.

In other words, LTDs and STDs can be considered the same thing. LTD is more general, and STD is more specific. LTDs arise from ANY risky behavior, and STDs arise from SPECIFIC risky behaviors.

And we can imagine that because STDs arise from specific zombie behaviors, there must exist alternative recovery behaviors that minimize the risk of STDs as follows:

ZOMBIE Behaviors	RECOVERY Behaviors
Zombie Seduction	TR Seduction
Multiple sex partners	Abstinence, contraception, monogamy
Injection drug use	Abstinence

We've now made a complete circle talking about LTDs and STDs. They are perfect companions for each other because they are part of the same problem. STDs and LTDs are caused by risk-taking behaviors. They can be avoided by adopting sensible behaviors.

The LTD concept fits with everything we've learned from STDs. It helps us talk more openly about risky eating behaviors, risky sexual behaviors, and risky drug use behaviors. It helps us resist pressure from family, from friends — from anyone.

The LTD concept should help you see the journey to recovery more clearly. It will guide you on your journey for the rest of your long and sensible life.

The CDC NEEDS to be ACTIVATED

We need our federal government to treat our LTD epidemic as seriously as outbreaks of Ebola, MERS, and HIV. Far more people are dying from LTDs than from infectious diseases. We need an agency like the Centers for Disease Control to coordinate all federal activities to fight LTDs.

The CDC currently coordinates local NCD efforts with their National Center for Chronic Disease Prevention and Health Promotion that adopts the lengthy acronym NCCDPHP.[211] And, they coordinate global NCD efforts with their Division of Global Health Protection that adopts the acronym DGHP.[212]

The CDC is taking some first steps with provocative messaging. They warn us our hearts may be older than our calendar ages.[213] This type of messaging fits perfectly with the philosophy of TR and LTDs.

But the CDC needs to take the provocative messaging up many more notches. LTDs are infectious. They're spreading. They're killing us.

Let's imagine what it might look like if the CDC builds up a massive LTD campaign modeled upon their STD campaign.

Media access. They could build media-accessible headquarters with giant screens tracking the LTD, STD, viral, and microbial epidemics. They could report quarterly deaths from the LTD epidemic alongside new viral, microbial, and STD cases. They could broadcast medical images of LTD-affected organs as the images come in from field clinics.

Media strategy. They could engage health professionals, the public, and, most importantly, our entertainment industry.

Zombie shows. The CDC is at the center of zombie apocalypse movies and TV shows. They could provide CDC scientists as consultants. They could help with scripts and special effects. They could help develop more plausible LTD and STD backstories.

Dramatic shows. The CDC could consult for medical and crime dramas too.

Competition shows. The CDC could help with reality TV shows based on cooking, adventure, and romance competition. Their scientists could help eliminate contestants based on LTD-

---

211   CDC website. **Chronic Disease Prevention and Health Promotion.** Accessed 2016. *cdc.gov/chronicdisease*

212   CDC website. **Global Health Protection and Security.** Accessed 2016. *cdc.gov/globalhealth/healthprotection/ncd*

213   CDC website. **Vital Signs>Topics Covered>Cardiovascular Diseases>Heart Age.** Accessed 2016. *cdc.gov/vitalsigns/heartage*

promoting food choices, leisure choices, and sexual choices.

Judging panel. Every new reality TV show tries to get an edge on its competition. What could be a better edge than an actual CDC scientist on a judging panel? The CDC scientists could show off their latest medical images from the field to explain their judging decisions.

Recruiting competition. The CDC could prepare for their LTD media effort by recruiting scientists who are smart and telegenic. The recruiting effort could be done as a reality TV show contest. The young scientist may participate in events such as male and female fitness competitions, food preparation competitions, and debates about LTD mechanisms and mitigation strategies.

The possibilities are endless. We just need the CDC to get activated.

ZOMBIE INC.

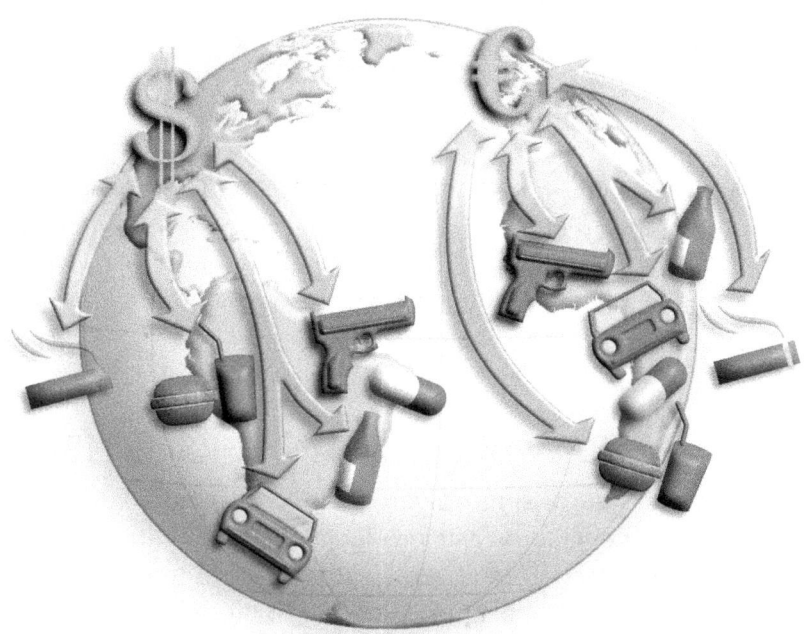

Zombie Inc. prospers while our health and the environment languishes.

Multinational corporations help shape the Western lifestyle by marketing unhealthy commodities such as tobacco, alcohol, junk food, and gasoline. These corporations encourage zombie behaviors that erode our personal health and the health of the environment. These corporations generate profits from our zombie behaviors. TR represents these corporations as Zombie Inc. and it represents their profits as zombie profits.

In this chapter, we examine the following topics:
- *Zombie profits versus health.*
- *The Lancet NCD Action Group.*
- *Zombie profits without borders.*
- *Zombie profits versus government.*

- *Zombie profits win free speech rights.*
- *"Made in USA" versus "Made in China"*
- *Hiding behind "Responsible use"*
- *Zombie profits versus science.*
- *Zombie profits versus the environment.*
- *Zombie profit heaven on Earth.*
- *Zombie profits versus regulators.*
- *Review.*
- *Imagine.*

Advisory. This chapter is partly intended to inspire stronger health and safety regulations. To this end, it gets more politically charged than other chapters. If you feel strongly that our government is the problem and that our free market is the solution, then you may want to skip this chapter entirely.

ZOMBIE PROFITS VERSUS HEALTH

Zombie Inc. has surprising power over us. It manufactures zombie viruses that entice us to buy its products. It disseminates these viruses through advertisements. It seduces us to indulge and overuse its unhealthy products. It fuels the epidemic of lifestyle transmitted disease.

Zombie Inc. goes by different names such as:

- Big Tobacco[**214**]
- Big Alcohol[**215**]
- Big Food[**216**]
- Big Soda[**217**]
- Big Oil[**218**]
- Big Coal[**219**]

214 Wikipedia. **Big Tobacco.** Accessed 2016. *en.wikipedia.org/wiki/Big_Tobacco*

215 Moodie AR. **Big alcohol: the vector of an industrial epidemic.** Addiction. 2014 Apr;109(4):525-6. *pubmed.gov/24605954*

216 PLOS Collections. **PLoS Medicine Series on Big Food.** Accessed 2016. *ploscollections.org/article/browseIssue.action?issue=info:doi/10.1371/issue.pcol.v07.i17*

217 Wikipedia. **Big Soda.** Accessed 2016. *en.wikipedia.org/wiki/Big_soda*

218 Wikipedia. **Big Oil.** Accessed 2016. *en.wikipedia.org/wiki/Big_Oil*

219 Wikipedia. **Big Coal: The Dirty Secret Behind America's Energy Future.** Accessed 2016. *en.wikipedia.org/wiki/Big_Coal:_The_Dirty_*

- Big Media[**220**]
- handgun dealers[**221**]
- drug dealers[**222**]

We're all familiar with Zombie Inc. because we enjoy its products, though we know we shouldn't enjoy them too often. We enjoy the advertisements, mascots, and brands related to its products. Its brands form our Western culture. Its products form our Western lifestyle.

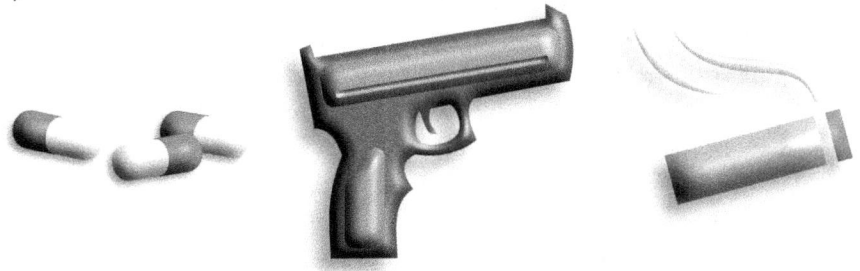

Zombie Inc. generates tremendous profits which are very different from normal profits. Zombie profits are constrained by government regulations. When government regulations are strong, zombie profits decrease. When government regulations are weak, zombie profits increase.

To increase zombie profits, Zombie Inc. is driven to weaken government regulations and weaken government itself. It manufactures zombie viruses to manipulate the political environment. It disseminates these viruses through political advertising and by financing pro-business and anti-regulation politicians.

Free trade agreements between countries expand globalization and weaken the power of developing countries to regulate Zombie Inc. Globalization strengthens the power of Zombie Inc. and fuels the widening epidemic of lifestyle transmitted diseases.

Secret_Behind_America%27s_Energy_Future

220 Wikipedia. **Media conglomerate.** Accessed 2016. *en.wikipedia.org/wiki/Media_conglomerate*

221 Wikipedia. **Small arms trade.** Accessed 2016. *en.wikipedia.org/wiki/Small_arms_trade*

222 Wikipedia. **Illegal drug trade.** Accessed 2016. *en.wikipedia.org/wiki/Illegal_drug_trade*

THE LANCET NCD ACTION GROUP

Brave health researchers with the Lancet NCD Action Group analyze how the tobacco, alcohol, processed food, and drink industries contribute to the spread of non-communicable diseases (NCDs). [**223**] They refer to Zombie Inc. as UNHEALTHY COMMODITIES INDUSTRIES. Their blunt analysis is such a breakthrough in health research that TR dedicates this chapter to their ongoing efforts.

In this chapter, we'll refer to NCDs as LTDs most of the time. And, we'll refer to the Unhealthy Commodities Industries as Zombie Inc. most of the time. We'll switch back and forth between these naming schemes.

We'll also refer to the Lancet NCD Action Group by an acronym: the Lancet NAG. This acronym and this citation [**Lancet NAG**] will appear often because this entire chapter is hereby dedicated to studying the Lancet "NAG" the Unhealthy Commodity Industries.

ZOMBIE PROFITS WITHOUT BORDERS

The Lancet NAGs the Unhealthy Commodity Industries for spreading the epidemic of NCDs across borders and for causing widespread deaths around the world. The tobacco industry causes 6 million NCD deaths every year. The alcohol industry causes 5 million NCD deaths every year. The processed food and drink industries cause 18 million NCD deaths every year as a result of obesity, high blood sugar, high blood pressure, and high cholesterol.[**Lancet NAG**]

The Lancet NAGs the Unhealthy Commodity Industries about how they use globalization, free-trade agreements, and developing markets to fuel growth. These companies are typically enormous multinational corporations that span markets across the globe. The ten largest alcohol producers control 66% of the global market. The two largest soft drink companies control 50% of the global market. The ten largest food companies control 50% of U.S. food sales but only 15% of global food sales. These companies view the sales to

223 Moodie R, Stuckler D, Monteiro C, Sheron N, Neal B, Thamarangsi T, Lincoln P, Casswell S; Lancet NCD Action Group. **Profits and pandemics: prevention of harmful effects of tobacco, alcohol, and ultra-processed food and drink industries.** Lancet. 2013 Feb 23;381(9867): 670-9. *pubmed.gov/23410611*

developing markets as a large growth opportunity.[**Lancet NAG**]

In the developing country, a free trade agreement with the U.S. causes market deregulation, undermines local control, and increases unhealthy commodity sales. For instance, soft drink sales typically increase by 63%.[**224**]

The Lancet NAGs the Unhealthy Commodity Industries on how they follow each other into developing markets and learn each others' techniques. Tobacco and alcohol industries penetrate first. Soda and food industries follow. All unhealthy commodities use common tactics. The sales of tobacco are a leading indicator for sales of other NCD-transmitting products. Across local markets, tobacco sales correlate with alcohol, soft drink, and processed food sales. Consumption of big food and big soda is increasing fastest in lower-middle income countries. Obesity is rising simultaneously.[**Lancet NAG**]

ZOMBIE PROFITS VERSUS GOVERNMENT

Zombie profits are unique because they are limited by government regulations more than profits from typical corporations. The government regulates the sales and promotion of Zombie Inc. products to protect us from over-using and abusing its products and to protect our kids from underage use.

Unfortunately, Zombie Inc. is in a bind. As a corporation, it has a FIDUCIARY DUTY on behalf of its shareholders to maximize zombie profits.[**225**] At the same time, it has a LEGAL DUTY to follow government regulations.

But, Zombie Inc. has NO OBLIGATION to go out of its way to support our long-term health, our environment, and government regulations — or to even support our government. Its loyalty to zombie profits comes first.

In fact, Zombie Inc. has a fiduciary duty to increase zombie profits, which means it must do what it can to weaken government regulations, to weaken government, and to create a political climate

---

224 Stuckler D, McKee M, Ebrahim S, Basu S. **Manufacturing epidemics: the role of global producers in increased consumption of unhealthy commodities including processed foods, alcohol, and tobacco.** PLoS Med. 2012;9(6):e1001235. *pubmed.gov/22745605*

225 Wikipedia. **Fiduciary.** Accessed 2016. *en.wikipedia.org/wiki/ Fiduciary*

that is hostile to government regulations. Once again, its loyalty to zombie profits comes before our long-term health, our environment, our government regulations, and our government.

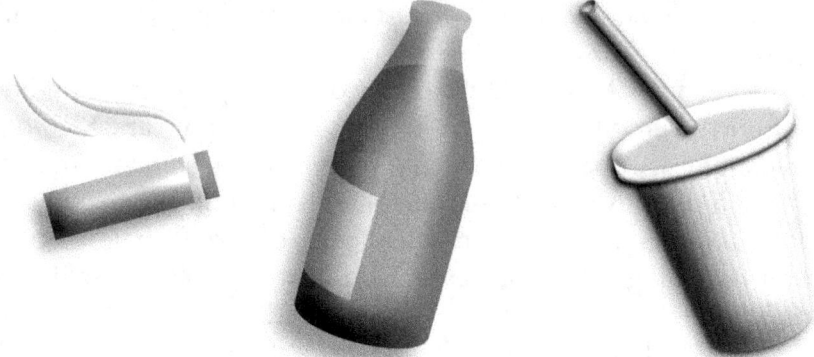

The Lancet NAG bravely shines a spotlight on the political activities of the Unhealthy Commodity Industries. The Lancet NAGs them for using its profits to weaken government regulations and to weaken the government.[**Lancet NAG**] In the battle of zombie profits versus government, zombie profits have a surprising advantage.

Zombie Inc. patiently executes a multi-year business plan to invest zombie profits in weakening government regulations and in weakening government. It finances the political campaigns of pro-business and anti-government politicians. It persuades us as voters to oppose government regulations.

Most importantly, Zombie Inc. changes the political climate by investing zombie profits into the manufacture and dissemination of the following zombie viruses:

Nanny state virus. This zombie virus causes us zombies to oppose public health measures. This virus celebrates individual responsibility rather than government regulations.[**226**]

Big government virus. This zombie virus causes us zombies to oppose government regulations.[**227**]

Government waste virus. This zombie virus causes us zombies to overestimate government "waste, fraud, and abuse." We oppose government use of tax revenue, and we demand revenue be re-

226 Wikipedia. **Nanny state.** Accessed 2016. *en.wikipedia.org/wiki/Nanny_state*

227 Wikipedia. **Big government.** Accessed 2016. *en.wikipedia.org/wiki/Big_government*

turned to taxpayers in the form of tax cuts.[228]

Tax cut stimulus virus. This zombie virus causes us zombies to believe tax cuts spur economic growth. We are led to believe CUTTING taxes actually brings in MORE tax revenue.[229]

Starve the beast virus. This zombie virus causes us zombies to believe tax cuts cause the government to shrink in size. We are led to believe CUTTING taxes brings in LESS tax revenue and enforces LESS government spending.[230] This belief is completely inconsistent with the previous virus, yet we happily hold both viruses in our heads at the same time. This belief is also inconsistent with federal deficit spending and a growing federal debt.

Job creator virus. This zombie virus causes us zombies to revere corporations, executives, and the wealthy as if they are celebrities.[231]

Death tax virus. This zombie virus causes us zombies to defend wealthy children from inheritance taxes as if they are vulnerable and need our protection.[232] This virus almost brings tears to our eyes thinking about the plight of wealthy children having to pay enormous taxes to a big fat government.

It may not be obvious why Zombie Inc. promotes tax cut viruses. The Lancet NAG points out that when the government cuts taxes, it has less tax revenue, and it faces more difficulty enforcing regulations.[**Lancet NAG**] In the U.S., state governments must balance their budgets, and indeed, often reduce regulatory staff. On the other hand, the federal government routinely runs budget deficits and does not necessarily need to reduce regulatory staff.

However, over time, tax cuts eventually weaken the federal government. A weaker federal government gradually loosens regula-

228 Wikipedia. **Government_waste.** Accessed 2016. *en.wikipedia.org/wiki/Government_waste*

229 Wikipedia. **Supply-side economics.** Accessed 2016. *en.wikipedia.org/wiki/Supply-side_economics*

230 Wikipedia. **Starve the beast.** Accessed 2016. *en.wikipedia.org/wiki/Starve_the_beast*

231 Wikipedia. **Chief executive officer.** Accessed 2016. *en.wikipedia.org/wiki/Chief_executive_officer*

232 Wikipedia. **Estate tax in the United_States.** Accessed 2016. *en.wikipedia.org/wiki/Estate_tax_in_the_United_States*

tory authority over the Unhealthy Commodities Industries.[**Lancet NAG**] In the long run, zombie profits have a surprising advantage in the battle against government.

ZOMBIE PROFITS WIN FREE SPEECH RIGHTS

The U.S. citizen may notice that federal politics and campaigns have become increasingly bizarre. We witness politicians doing strange things that don't seem good for the country. We witness politicians behaving recklessly with the country's future. We don't realize we're actually witnessing an uptick in the ferocity of the battle of zombie profits versus government.

The U.S. Supreme Court recently granted zombie profits even greater power. It granted free speech rights to unlimited corporate spending in U.S. elections. Do you find this confusing? Most of us have a hard time equating free SPEECH with political SPENDING, but that's what the U.S Supreme Court did.

Citizens United V FEC. This U.S. Supreme Court case in 2010 challenged whether the Federal Elections Commission can limit campaign spending by corporations. In a partisan 5-4 split decision, the Supreme Court ruled against the FEC. The razor-thin partisan majority extended the First Amendment free speech rights of a U.S. citizen to the political spending of any corporation.[233]

In the Supreme Court ruling, the majority publicly states, "political SPENDING is a form of protected SPEECH under the First Amendment."[234] The majority reasoned that because a corporation is treated as a person in a court of law, then a corporation should have the same political free speech rights as a U.S. citizen. They breathed new life into a concept called corporate personhood. [235]

The Supreme Court majority turned the First Amendment com-

---

233 Wikipedia. **Citizens United v FEC.** Accessed 2016. *en.wikipedia.org/ wiki/Citizens_United_v._FEC*

234 SCOTUSblog. **Citizens United v. Federal Election Commission.** Accessed 2016. Supreme Court of the United States. *scotusblog.com/ case-files/cases/citizens-united-v-federal-election-commission*

235 Wikipedia. **Corporate personhood.** Accessed 2016. *en.wikipedia.org/ wiki/Corporate_personhood*

pletely upside-down. They forgot that the First Amendment was intended to protect the rights of the POWERLESS citizen. They granted First Amendment rights to POWERFUL multinational corporations whose power rivals that of small countries.

Social welfare corporation. Under current law, a public corporation can set up a shell corporation to handle all political activity. [**236**] Within government regulations, it's called a social welfare corporation, or a 501(c)(4). It has an innocuous name, but it has amazing powers.

A social welfare corporation can: maintain the secrecy of its donors; support or oppose a candidate for public office; lobby U.S. representatives and senators; run unlimited political advertising at any time during a primary campaign or a general election; run political advertising that is completely false because its donors are kept secret, and they don't suffer consequences.

The *Citizens United V FEC* decision in 2010 combined with the secrecy of the social welfare corporation create a powerful weapon for political influence. Wealthy corporations and wealthy individuals can now HIDE unlimited political spending. In 2006, BEFORE *Citizens United*, contributions to social welfare corporations totaled $5 million. In 2012, AFTER *Citizens United*, contributions totaled over $300 million, which is a 60-fold increase.[**237**]

Foreign influence. By granting First Amendment free speech rights to social welfare corporations, the Supreme Court is extending unlimited political influence to secret donors to these corporations. Consequently, any secret person or organization can establish a social welfare corporation and influence U.S. elections and the U.S. government. A social welfare corporation can be anonymously funded by: U.S. and foreign companies, U.S. and foreign billionaires, or even foreign governments.[**238**] There's no way to find out. Donors are anonymous.

A dollar from any source — domestic or foreign — now has

---

236 Wikipedia. **501(c) organization.** Accessed 2016. *en.wikipedia.org/wiki/501(c)_organization*

237 Wikipedia. **Citizens United v FEC.** Accessed 2016. *en.wikipedia.org/wiki/Citizens_United_v._FEC*

238 Mother Jones website. **Politics>How Secret Foreign Money Could Infiltrate US Elections.** Accessed 2016. *motherjones.com/politics/2012/08/foreign-dark-money-2012-election-nonprofit*

free speech rights better than a U.S. citizen because it is an anonymous dollar. The dollar can say or do anything. There are no consequences to its reputation. It's anonymous.

Freedom of false speech. The anonymous dollar can team up with 300 million other anonymous dollars and have more free speech rights than there are U.S. citizens eligible to vote. Anonymous dollars actually have freedom of ACCURATE speech and freedom of FALSE speech since there are no consequences to an anonymous donor for false speech. The U.S. citizen should be jealous and angry.

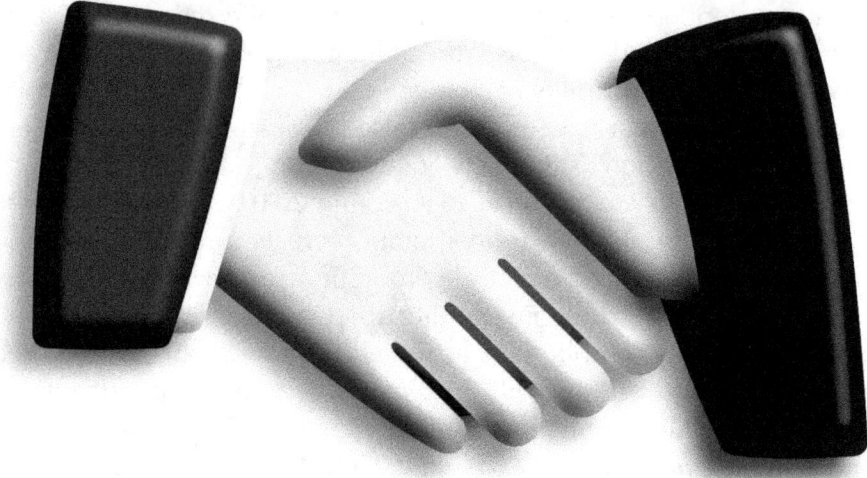

The Supreme Deal: Citizens United v FEC 2010

With their ruling on the case of *Citizens United V FEC*, the Supreme Court granted extraordinary powers to zombie profits and Zombie Inc. It gave Zombie Inc. an investment deal that it quite literally CANNOT refuse. Zombie Inc. would FAIL its fiduciary duty to its shareholders if it refuses the deal.

Once we understand the power of zombie profits, the 501(c)(4) social welfare corporation, and *Citizens United V FEC*, we can understand why each of us — including Zombie Inc. — is now held captive to unlimited corporate political spending.

- Zombie Inc. MUST invest zombie profits into U.S. political campaigns to reduce government regulations.
- Politicians MUST behave recklessly with our country's future to receive campaign support from Zombie Inc.
- U.S. citizens MUST accept increasingly bizarre political the-

atrics and election campaigns.

We can all thank the U.S. Supreme Court for the supreme investment deal it offered Zombie Inc.

"MADE IN USA" VERSUS "MADE IN CHINA"

The "Made in USA" label on a product — particularly on food — reassures us we can trust it. We need to consider thinking of the "Made in USA" label as a marketing brand.

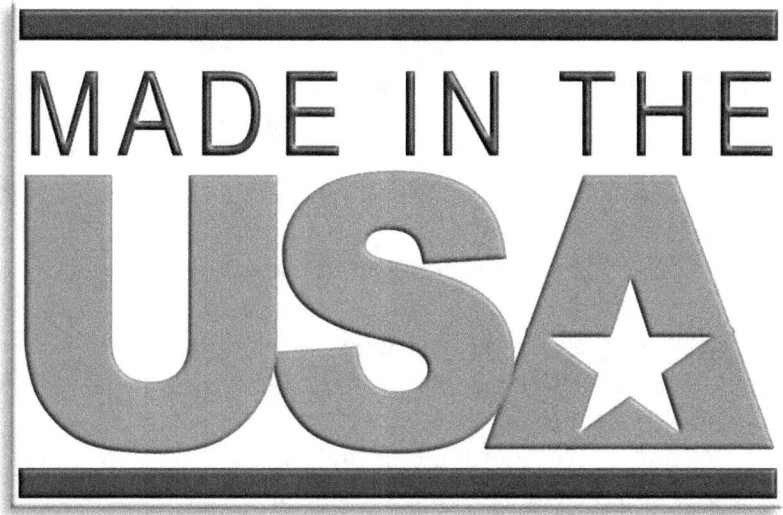

Government oversight strengthens the U.S.A. brand.

Consider who helps to strengthen the "Made in USA" brand. The U.S. government strengthens the brand with regulations to ensure that every company plays by the rules of health and safety. U.S. companies strengthen the brand when they play by the rules. Employees of U.S. companies strengthen the brand when they exercise their whistleblower protections. Investigative journalists strengthen the brand when they report on cheaters.

We should feel confident eating food with the "Made in USA" brand.

The "Made in China" label on a product should have a very different effect. It warns us we should beware of the product — especially when it's a food item or a toy our children might put in their mouths. Food safety incidents occur frequently in China.[239] For instance, in 2008, Chinese dairy companies spiked milk and infant formula with a toxic chemical to give the appearance it contained more protein. Around 300,000 infants were sickened, 50,000 infants required hospitalization, and six infants died.

Consider who helps to weaken the "Made in China" brand. The Chinese government weakens the brand because of multiple conflicts of interest. It maintains partial ownership of large businesses. It considers criticisms of its corporations as criticisms of itself. It has an intolerance for political dissent. It struggles to be open and honest with its public about health and safety. Chinese companies weaken the brand when they seek quick profits. Chinese workers are unable to strengthen the brand because they have no whistle-blower protections.

We should NOT feel confident eating food with the "Made in China" brand.

Most U.S. corporations understand the value of the "Made in USA" brand. They incorporate social responsibility into their business models to boost the value of their own brands.[240] These corporations embrace government oversight to ensure there's a safe and fair playing field to do business.

For instance, a U.S. airline corporation can truthfully claim that flying with a U.S. airline is as safe or safer than traveling by car. The U.S. airline industry relies on U.S. government oversight to maintain passenger safety. U.S. government oversight also ensures every U.S. airline plays by the same rules and operates in a safe manner.

Zombie Inc. is in a curious position where it can claim its products are safe for light use. It adheres to U.S. government regulations to make sure its products don't make us immediately sick. With light use, its products live up to the "Made in USA" brand quality.

But Zombie Inc. CANNOT claim its products are safe for heavy and long-term use. It CANNOT claim its products are safe for our kids to use. Such use erodes our health and the health of our environment.

---

239 Wikipedia. **Food safety incidents in China.** Accessed 2016. *en. wikipedia.org/wiki/Food_safety_incidents_in_China*

240 Wikipedia. **Corporate social responsibility.** Accessed 2016. *en. wikipedia.org/wiki/Corporate_social_responsibility*

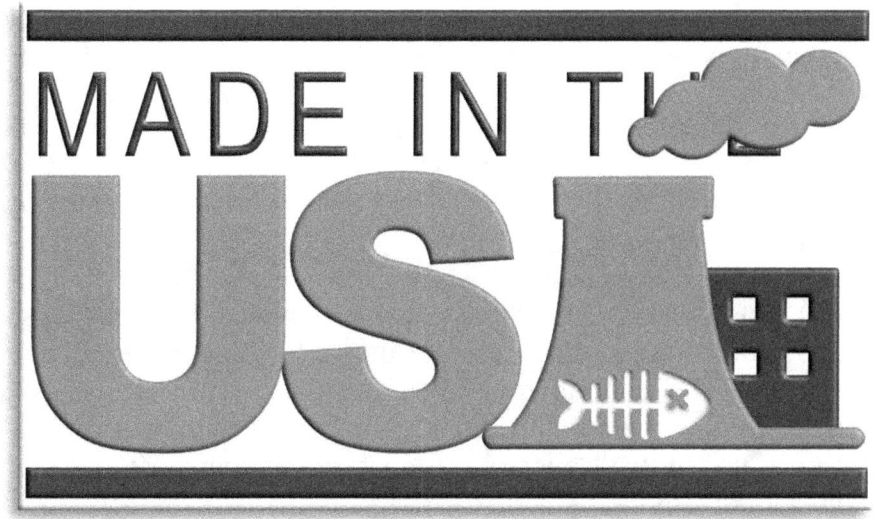

Zombie inc. misconduct weakens the U.S.A. brand.

When Zombie Inc. undermines our government oversight and it markets the heavy use, long-term use, or underage use of its products, it damages the "Made in USA" brand and makes it look like the "Made in China" brand.

HIDING BEHIND "RESPONSIBLE USE"

Zombie Inc. doesn't warn us in explicit terms about the health risks of heavy use or long-term use of its products. Instead, it advises us to exercise the "responsible use" of its products.

The responsible use claim is quite effective. It gives the impression that Zombie Inc. understands the meaning of responsible behavior. It's like a wink and a nod between Zombie Inc. and us.

The responsible use claim allows Zombie Inc. to use kid-friendly cartoon characters to advertise its products. The responsible use claim means its advertisements are intended for our kids, but the actual products are intended for us. It's like a wink and a nod between Zombie Inc. and our kids. And it's quite effective.

Marlboro cigarettes began using Joe Camel in 1988 to teach children about responsible use.[**241**] Within three years, medical re-

---

241 Wikipedia. **Joe Camel.** Accessed 2016. *en.wikipedia.org/wiki/Joe_Camel*

searchers found 91% of six-year-olds could recognize Joe Camel as a cigarette mascot — a rate of recognition as high as Disney mascots. Within the same period of time, Camel cigarette sales to children grew from 1% to 33% of total illegal sales. 33% of illegal sales is dramatic, but it's clearly less than the 91% rate of mascot recognition, so the remaining children clearly understood "responsible use" with the cartoon mascot.

Budweiser Beer uses a variety of kid-friendly mascots to teach about responsible use. Spuds MacKenzie appeared in 1987.[242] The Budweiser Frogs, also known as Bud, Weis, and Er, appeared in 1995.[243] They were followed by wise-cracking chameleons. Talking lizards now represent the brand. The talking animals don't drink the beer, they just talk about it, which is an important lesson to children about "responsible use."

Ronald McDonald teaches children about responsible use.[244] The clown moves a lot — an important lesson for children who may forget to exercise. The clown visits McDonald's restaurants but doesn't eat the food — another important lesson about "responsible use" for children.

Kellogg's maintains a portfolio of food mascots to teach children about "responsible use."[245] Their portfolio includes Toucan Sam, Tony the Tiger, Snap-Crackle-and-Pop, and the Keebler Elves. Every mascot is active and fit. None of them sits on a couch for prolonged periods. None is obese. None complains about high blood sugar, high insulin, or diabetes.

ZOMBIE PROFITS VERSUS SCIENCE

The Lancet NAGs the Unhealthy Commodity Industries for creating misleading health advocacy organizations.[**Lancet NAG**] Zombie

242 Wikipedia. **Spuds MacKenzie.** Accessed 2016. *en.wikipedia.org/wiki/ Spuds_MacKenzie*

243 Wikipedia. **Budweiser Frogs.** Accessed 2016. *en.wikipedia.org/wiki/ Budweiser_Frogs*

244 Wikipedia. **Ronald McDonald.** Accessed 2016. *en.wikipedia.org/ wiki/Ronald_McDonald*

245 Wikipedia. **Kellogg's.** Accessed 2016. *en.wikipedia.org/wiki/Kellogg %27s*

profits fund unhealthy commodity advocacy organizations which operate as follows:

- The unhealthy commodity advocacy organizations adopt names that — by coincidence — give the APPEARANCE of legitimate health advocacy organizations.
- They hire researchers to publish articles that — by coincidence — SUPPORT the unhealthy commodities.
- They fund outside researchers to publish articles that — by coincidence — are four to eight times more likely to conclude negligible health risks of unhealthy commodities, leading to public confusion.
- They commission reports that — by coincidence — resemble reports released by the World Health Organization, leading to public confusion.

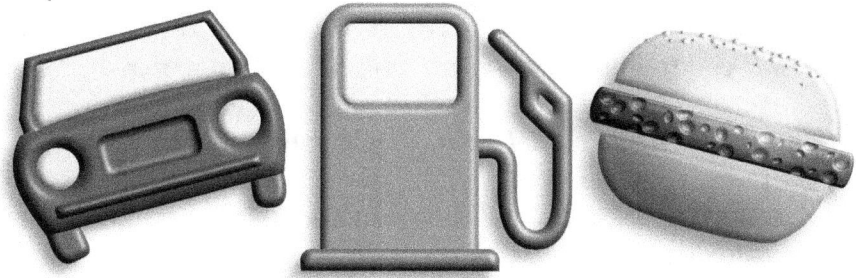

The unhealthy commodity advocacy organizations help contribute to the larger problem of distorting science to fit politics such as:[246]

- The tobacco industry disputes its role in cancer.[247]
- The energy industry disputes its role in global warming.[248]
- The coal industry disputes its role in polluting the air, water, and soil.[249]

246 Wikipedia. **Politicization of science.** Accessed 2016. *en.wikipedia. org/wiki/Politicization_of_science*

247 Wikipedia. **Tobacco politics.** Accessed 2016. *en.wikipedia.org/wiki/ Tobacco_politics*

248 Wikipedia. **Climate change denial.** Accessed 2016. *en.wikipedia.org/ wiki/Climate_change_denial*

249 Wikipedia. **Environmental impact of the coal industry.** Accessed 2016.   *en.wikipedia.org/wiki/Environmental_impact_of_the_coal_ industry*

- The agricultural industry disputes its role in algae blooms and dead fish zones in lakes and oceans.[250]

ZOMBIE PROFITS VERSUS THE ENVIRONMENT

Zombie profits are also constrained by government regulations that protect the environment, such as endangered species, clean air, clean water, and clean soil.

Profits from other corporations don't have this conflict. Other corporations embrace environmental health within their business models.[251] They try, for instance, to reduce their landfill waste, their energy consumption, and their carbon footprint.

But Zombie Inc. has a different business model. It uses zombie profits to manufacture and disseminate the following zombie viruses:

Anti-environmentalism virus. This zombie virus causes us zombies to virulently oppose environmental conservation.[252]

Climate change denial virus. This zombie virus causes us zombies to virulently oppose environmental science.[253] This virus causes us zombies to deny the human contribution to atmospheric carbon dioxide and climate change.

Abolish the EPA virus. This zombie virus causes us zombies to virulently oppose the Environmental Protection Agency.[254] This virus encourages politicians to block regulations by the Environmental Protection Agency and to threaten to shut it down. This virus makes us all forget that the EPA was created by Richard Nixon to protect human health and the environment. It makes us all forget

250 Wikipedia. **Dead zone (ecology).** Accessed 2016. *en.wikipedia.org/wiki/Dead_zone_(ecology)*

251 Wikipedia. **Sustainable business.** Accessed 2016. *en.wikipedia.org/wiki/Sustainable_business*

252 Wikipedia. **Anti-environmentalism.** Accessed 2016. *en.wikipedia.org/wiki/Anti-environmentalism*

253 Wikipedia. **Climate change denial.** Accessed 2016. *en.wikipedia.org/wiki/Climate_change_denial*

254 Wikipedia. **U.S. Environmental Protection Agency.** Accessed 2016. *en.wikipedia.org/wiki/United_States_Environmental_Protection_Agency*

that the EPA protects us and our children from polluting corporations.

Zombie Inc. spreads these viruses with anonymously-funded social welfare corporations that in turn fund all their political lobbying, political advertising, and voter mobilization campaigns.

ZOMBIE PROFIT HEAVEN ON EARTH

Let's imagine what life in the U.S. would be like without the EPA. Imagine living in a country where Unhealthy Commodity Industries can boost profits without health regulation, safety regulation, and environmental regulation. Imagine living in ZOMBIE PROFIT HEAVEN.

Well, we're in luck. We don't have to imagine too hard. Such a place exists. China.

Industries in China can pollute freely to boost profits. They have the government on their side. Residents can complain, but it doesn't matter. The government doesn't listen to the residents. The government listens to profits. China is ZOMBIE PROFIT HEAVEN on Earth.

China also happens to be ENVIRONMENTAL HELL on Earth. China suffers the kind of pollution that U.S. residents cannot comprehend.[255] Chinese air, water, and soil set new records of toxicity every year.

- Coal combustion emits particulate matter that causes asthma, bronchitis, shortness of breath, painful breathing, lung cancer, and cardiovascular disease.
- Major cities in China are constantly covered in a toxic gray shroud.
- In 2007, a draft World Bank report on China stated: toxic urban air causes over 350,000 premature deaths each year; toxic indoor air causes another 300,000 premature deaths each year; toxic drinking water causes 60,000 premature deaths each year.

---

255   Wikipedia. **Pollution in China.** Accessed 2016. *en.wikipedia.org/wiki/Pollution_in_China*

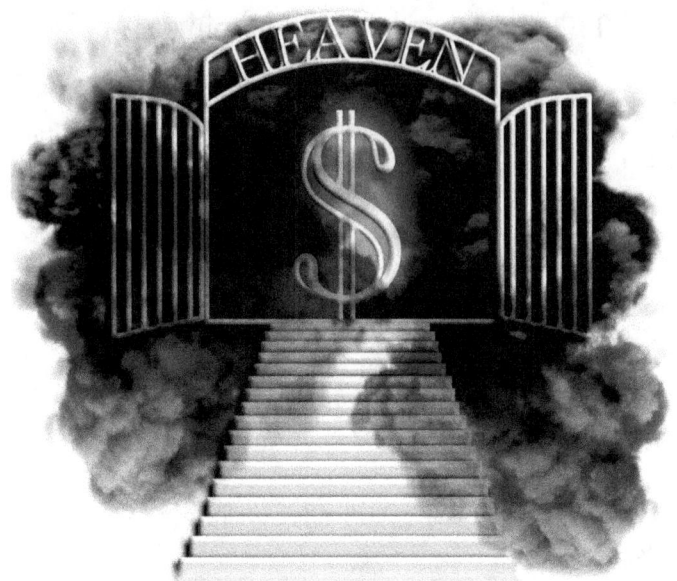

Zombie profit heaven on earth.

- In 2013, record smog levels in northeastern China reached an all-time high.[**256**] Visibility dropped to 160 feet. Airports and schools were closed. The particulate levels not only exceeded World Health Organization recommended levels, they exceeded them by a factor of 50 — which as a percentage is 5,000%.
- Air pollution has reduced the life expectancy in northern China by 5.5 years.
- In 2013, China set a grim new record with the youngest person to die of lung cancer — an 8-year-old girl.

ZOMBIE PROFITS VERSUS REGULATORS

The Lancet NAGs the Unhealthy Commodity Industries about how they regularly deceive government regulators.[**Lancet NAG**] The industries routinely create products designed to appear more healthy. These products help the industry either evade or delay regulatory action. Here are examples:

The tobacco industry deceived government regulators with the light cigarette. This cigarette had invisibly small holes to allow air to

---

256 Wikipedia. **2013 Northeastern China smog.** Accessed 2016. *en. wikipedia.org/wiki/2013_Northeastern_China_smog*

decrease the concentration of smoke when being tested by government regulators. But, when being squeezed by the fingers of an actual smoker, the holes would close shut, increasing the concentration of smoke.[257] The invisible holes deceived government regulators into believing the light cigarette was a safer cigarette.

The automobile industry deceived government regulators with the "clean diesel" engine. This engine would automatically decrease its tailpipe emissions when being tested in an emissions facility. But, it would increase its tailpipe emissions to get better performance when being driven on the road.[258] This automatic adjustment of tailpipe emissions was designed to deceive government regulators into believing the "clean diesel" engine was good for the environment.

The soft drink industry markets sports drinks that appear to be more healthy alternatives to regular soda. Sports drinks are marketed as drinks for athleticism. Sports drinks technically have fewer sugar calories per ounce compared to regular soda, but they are still sugar-sweetened and derive most of their calories from sugar.[259]

The processed food industry markets reduced salt, reduced trans fat, and reduced calorie products that appear to be more healthy alternatives to regular convenience foods. These products still derive their calories from refined sugars, grains, and fats. They still fail to deliver nutrition that is anything close to that of fresh fruits and vegetables.[260]

257 Wikipedia. **Lights (cigarette_type).** Accessed 2016. *en.wikipedia.org/ wiki/Lights_(cigarette_type)*

258 Wikipedia. **Volkswagen emissions scandal.** Accessed 2016. *en. wikipedia.org/wiki/Volkswagen_emissions_scandal*

259 Wikipedia. **Sports drink.** Accessed 2016. *en.wikipedia.org/wiki/ Sports_drink*

260 Wikipedia. **Diet food.** Accessed 2016. *en.wikipedia.org/wiki/Diet_ food*

CHAPTER NINE REVIEW

Zombie inc. This fictitious company represents every corporation that sells an Unhealthy Commodity. It makes profits by selling products that erode our long term health and the health of the environment. It makes more profits when we overuse its products. It makes more profits when it recruits kids to use its products.

Zombie profits. These profits from Zombie Inc. are surprisingly powerful. In order to increase zombie profits, Zombie Inc. must do things that typical corporations would find objectionable. These profits corrode our health, the environment, government regulations, and even the government itself.

Government regulations. These regulations protect us — and especially our kids — from the excessive promotion of unhealthy products. These regulations limit the profits of Zombie Inc.

Citizens United V FEC. This Supreme Court decision in 2010 removed most campaign advertising limits and campaign spending limits for corporations.

Corporate free speech. The Supreme Court granted free speech rights to political spending by corporations. A corporation can broadcast political attack ads anytime — even on the day of an election. A corporation can secretly fund political attack ads by creating a corporate social welfare organization that keeps its donors anonymous.

Corporate personhood. The Supreme Court expanded the personhood rights of corporations when granting them free speech rights in the form of unlimited political spending in their 2010 decision on *Citizens United v FEC*.

Corporate welfare. Corporations can create a 501(c)(4) SOCIAL WELFARE CORPORATION to manage all their political activities. The donors to the social welfare corporation are kept anonymous. The social welfare corporation can then run political attack ads that do not actually have to be accurate because all donors are secret and free from repercussions.

Corporate free trade. Corporations help governments negotiate free trade agreements between nations. These agreements remove local government control over health and environmental regulations.

CHAPTER NINE IMAGINE

In the case of *Citizens United v FEC* in 2010, the U.S. Supreme Court ruled that "political SPENDING is a form of protected SPEECH under the First Amendment."[**261**] The Supreme Court stated that corporate free speech requires both the free flow of ideas AND the free flow of money.

Prior to this decision, corporations could freely express their political speech using press releases and interviews with the media. But corporations were sometimes ignored by the media. A corporation could have done what other powerless people do and start a hunger strike or walk across the United States by foot. Corporations have always had free speech rights to do the things the rest of us powerless people need to do to get attention.

But after *Citizens United*, corporations can now freely spend unlimited sums of money on advertising campaigns to express their political opinions. They can also secretly fund social welfare corporations to freely express false opinions. Very few U.S. citizens have this kind of wealth and power.

Imagine the day when the U.S. Supreme Court realizes that it really dropped the ball in its ruling on *Citizens United*. It missed a crucial opportunity to grant free speech rights to ALL FORMS OF SPENDING. Just like corporate free speech, a free market also requires the free flow of ideas AND the free flow of money. Imagine when the Supreme Court rules that "ANY spending is a form of protected speech under the First Amendment."

Such a ruling would free corporations from government regulations on their marketing speech. Zombie Inc. would be free to make any marketing claim anytime, anywhere, to anyone — including our kids. Zombie Inc. would be one step closer to zombie profit heaven on Earth.

Such a ruling would free corporations from having to hide behind secretly funded social welfare corporations. Zombie Inc. would be free to disseminate its anti-regulation zombie viruses at the same time it markets its own products.

Zombie Inc. would be free to create an integrated marketing

---

261 SCOTUSblog. **Citizens United v. Federal Election Commission.** Accessed 2016. Supreme Court of the United States. *scotusblog. com/case-files/cases/citizens-united-v-federal-election-commission*

campaign that simultaneously infects us with two kinds of zombie viruses — ones that undermine our personal self-regulation AND ones that undermine government regulations. Zombie Inc. would be two steps closer to zombie profit heaven on Earth.

ZOMBIE PROFITS VERSUS OUR HEALTH

Let's imagine how integrated zombie virus marketing will sound for products that directly affect our personal health.

"For a limited time, every pack of Marlboro Dad comes with a free sample of Marlboro Kid. It is bubble-gum flavored and low nicotine. You and your little cowboy can spend some quality time … in Marlboro country."

"For every 44-ounce Super Big Gulp sold, we make a donation to STOP THE DIABETES HOAX Political Action Committee. Help us build a future without the DIABETES HOAX hanging over the heads of our children."

"Every time you carry our BPA-ENRICHED water bottle, you express how you feel about government regulations. Act now, and you'll get a free 'Keep your hands off my Bisphenol-A' T-shirt and an adult-sized pacifier."

"For a limited time, every 40-ounce bottle of Olde English 800 Malt Liquor comes with a free sample of Olde English 800 Malt Lickers. They're bottle-shaped lollipops. The more you lick 'em, the closer you get to the surprise inside. Share some Malt Lickers with your little guy … it is 40 ounces of pure pleasure."

"Bring the kids with you to the Sizzlin' Sunless Tanning Center. The kids can play in our new Sizzlin' Fun House and Sizzlin' Tube Slide where every surface is UV emitting. And you can take a long nap in our sound-proof Sizzlin' Sleep Capsule. Here at Sizzlin' Sunless, 'Time flies, skin fries, and you won't believe your eyes'™."

"For every new prescription you bring to the BACK of our drug store, we give you a pack of store-brand cigarettes at the FRONT of the drug store. Light one up on us … at the corner of happy & healthy."

ZOMBIE PROFITS VERSUS the ENVIRONMENT

Let's imagine how integrated zombie virus marketing will sound for products that directly affect the health of our environment.

"Five cents of every gallon goes toward fighting environmental regulation. Earn a free car wash if you join any one of our fake consumer anti-regulation groups such as California Drivers Alliance or Fed Up at the Pump."[262]

"Every 100% beef burger you purchase provides another dose of human-grade antibiotics to our cows. Come celebrate our newest antibiotic-resistant bacteria called livestock associated methicillin-resistant Staphylococcus aureus,[263] aka flesh-eating bacteria. [264] In commemoration, we proudly present our flesh-eating bacteria burger. The meat simply melts in your mouth. It's to die for."

"Our turbo-diesel engine helps you out-smart government regulators. When it detects a smog check, it REDUCES pollution to appear as clean as a gasoline engine. When it detects a merge onto the highway, it BOOSTS pollution to appear as powerful as a rocket engine."[265]

"Our chewing tobacco helps you INCREASE your carbon footprint, one spatter at a time."

"Our gasoline is sourced from certified fracking operations. It means you're helping us turn bedrock and groundwater into fracking fudge. And you're helping us

262 Wikipedia. **Western States Petroleum Association.** Accessed 2016. *en.wikipedia.org/wiki/Western_States_Petroleum_Associa tion*

263 Wikipedia. **Methicillin-resistant Staphylococcus aureus.** Accessed 2016. *en.wikipedia.org/wiki/Methicillin-resistant_Staphylococcus_ aureus*

264 Wikipedia. **Necrotizing fasciitis.** Accessed 2016. *en.wikipedia. org/wiki/Necrotizing_fasciitis*

265 Wikipedia. **Volkswagen emissions scandal.** Accessed 2016. *en. wikipedia.org/wiki/Volkswagen_emissions_scandal*

turn sleepy hamlets into seismic hot spots."[266]

"For every double-double cheeseburger, we donate manure run-off to a local river or lake. With your help, we can make news with the next big algae bloom and fish kill."[267]

"Your new heavy-duty diesel-powered truck is rolling-coal ready. A $1,999 conversion kit turns your truck into a smoke-breathing dragon. No tree-hugger in an electric car, on a bike, or on the sidewalk will be safe from your toxic cloud. They'll wish they never tried to save the environment after you smoke 'em good."[268]

266 Wikipedia. **Environmental impact of hydraulic fracturing.** Accessed 2016. *en.wikipedia.org/wiki/Environmental_impact_of_hydraulic_fracturing*

267 Wikipedia. **Algal bloom.** Accessed 2016. *en.wikipedia.org/wiki/Algal_bloom*

268 Wikipedia. **Rolling coal.** Accessed 2016. *en.wikipedia.org/wiki/Rolling_coal*

CHAPTER TEN
EXPLORING YOUTHFUL COMMUNITIES

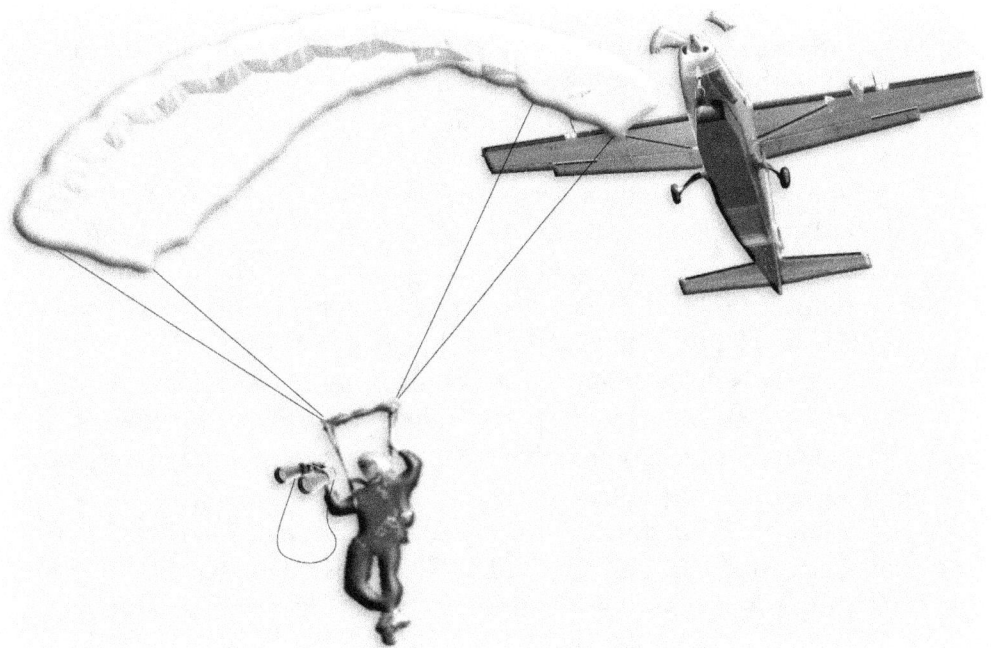

The journey to recovery seeks wisdom in youthful communities.

We now turn our attention to communities associated with exceptional youthfulness and longevity. These communities are scattered around the globe. Each community has its unique culture, lifestyle, and diet that resist aging and LTDs.

These communities flourished before globalization when the influence of Zombie Inc. was weak. These communities are now disappearing as globalization and Zombie Inc. become pervasive.

In this chapter, we examine the following topics:

- *Foods in the Blue Zones.*
- *Beans fuel the Blue Zones.*
- *Beans stimulate a dietary movement.*
- *Blue Zone special ops.*
- *Blue Zone undercover.*

- *A big shout out.*
- *Review.*
- *Imagine.*

FOODS IN THE BLUE ZONES

Italian demographers began a trend of referring to communities associated with exceptional longevity as Blue Zones. These demographers originally focused their attention on the Mediterranean community of Sardinia, Italy.[**269**]

Explorer Dan Buettner successfully popularizes the work of the Italian demographers with his series of books about Blue Zones. Buettner teams up with National Geographic to explore Sardinia, Italy, followed by Ikaria, Greece and other parts of world with communities associated with exceptional longevity.[**270**]

Buettner is not a scientist. He's an explorer. And he's a communicator. He has successfully popularized the study of healthy lifestyles. His ability to communicate the demography research to the general public is inspiring.

In honor of Buettner's inspiring work, TR creates an imaginary character called IMAGINARY BUETTNER. This character should not be confused with the real Buettner. Imaginary Buettner is an over-the-top explorer who lets us have some fun with the idea of exploring the globe and seeking wisdom from youthful communities.

Real Buettner and the demographers are in a race against the clock to study these youthful communities. Over time, fewer Blue Zone community members practice their traditional diets. The Blue Zone communities become contaminated by globalization, Zombie Inc., and the Western diet. These communities are in various stages of succumbing to the same LTDs and the same biological aging as the rest of us.

So far, demographers have collected a short list of traditional diets that resist biological aging and LTDs. They are trying to docu-

---

269 Poulain M, Pes GM, Grasland C, Carru C, Ferrucci L, Baggio G, Franceschi C, Deiana L. **Identification of a geographic area characterized by extreme longevity in the Sardinia island: the AKEA study.** Exp Gerontol. 2004 Sep;39(9):1423-9. *pubmed.gov/15489066*

270 Wikipedia. **Blue Zone.** Accessed 2016. *en.wikipedia.org/wiki/Blue_Zone*

ment these traditional diets before they completely disappear.

The Mediterranean Diet

Buettner and the Blue Zone team study two locations that incorporate the Mediterranean diet: Sardinia, Italy and Ikaria, Greece. The Mediterranean diet shows health benefits across many studies.[271] Compared to the Western diet, it contains less red meat and more whole fruits, whole vegetables, olive oil, whole grains, and fish.

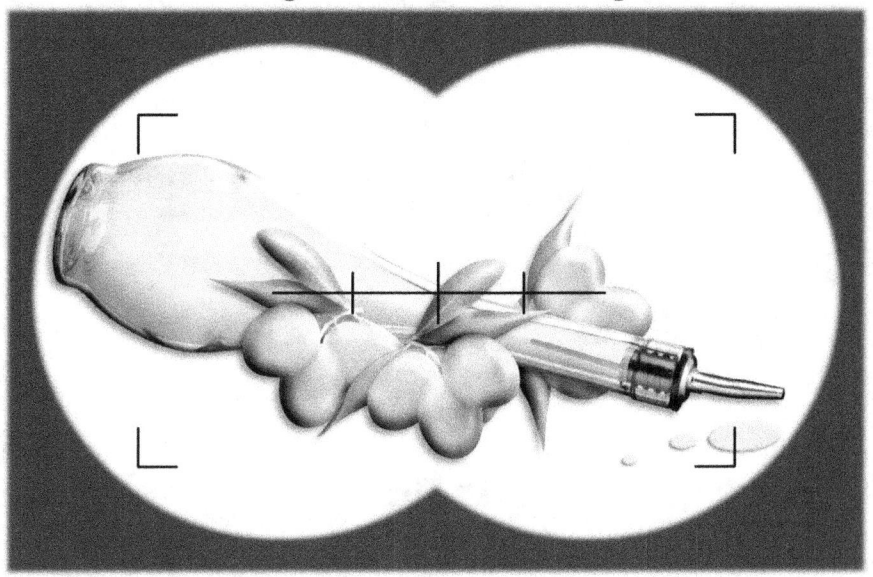

Imaginary Buettner observes olive oil in the Mediterranean diet.

The Mediterranean diet is a great option for people who prefer a mild change to their diets. On the upside, it inspires us to associate our meals with a beautiful part of the world rich in history. On the downside, it recommends some foods that the Gatherer diet identifies as snack foods.

The Rural Chinese Diet

The rural Chinese diet shows health benefits in the China-Cornell-Oxford Project, popularized by the book *The China Study* written by T. Colin Campbell.[272] The diet looks vegetarian and veg-

271 Wikipedia. **Mediterranean diet.** Accessed 2016. *en.wikipedia.org/wiki/Mediterranean_diet*

272 Wikipedia. **The China Study.** Accessed 2016. *en.wikipedia.org/wiki/The_China_Study*

an.

Despite the popularity of *The China Study* book, very few Westerners claim to follow the rural Chinese diet. Readers become inspired to experiment with vegetarianism and veganism, but they don't call their diet the rural Chinese diet. Perhaps readers are discouraged by the current health image of China, its food safety scandals, and its environmental pollution.

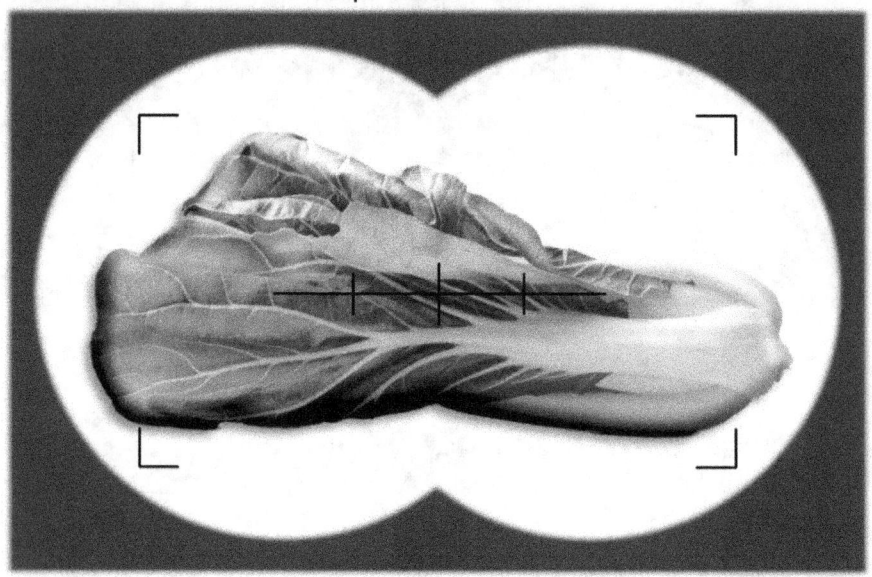

Imaginary Buettner observes bok choy in the rural Chinese diet.

The Okinawa Diet

Buettner and the Blue Zone team include the Japanese island of Okinawa as a longevity hotspot. The Okinawa diet shows longevity benefits in this island community in Japan.[273] The traditional Okinawa diet includes fruits and vegetables, occasional fish and pork, and very little rice or wheat.

The Okinawa diet is interesting because it relies on the sweet potato — a purple-flesh variety — which contributes nearly 70% of total calories. This diet could be considered the sweet potato diet.

If you love sweet potato, then this diet gives you permission to experiment and indulge.

---

273 Wikipedia. **Okinawa diet.** Accessed 2016. *en.wikipedia.org/wiki/Okinawa_diet*

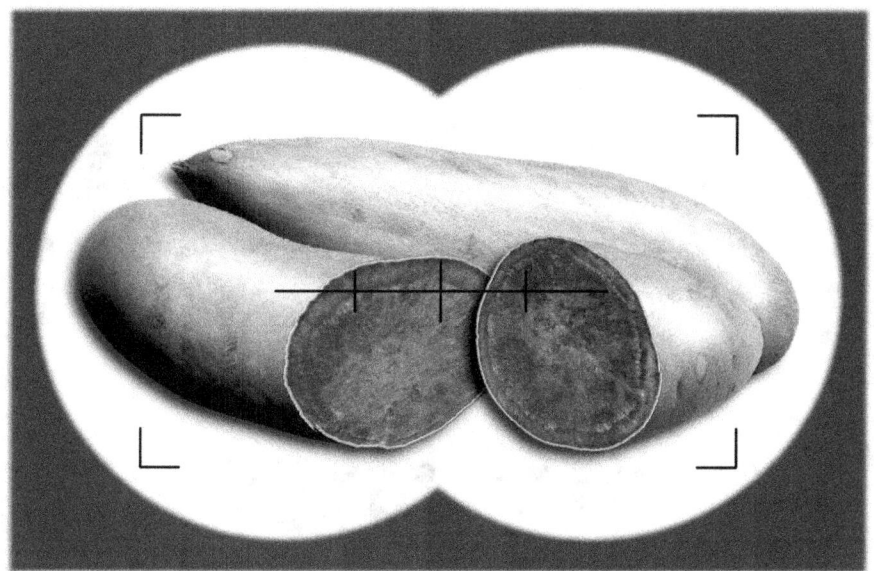

Imaginary Buettner observes the Okinawan purple sweet potato.

BEANS FUEL THE BLUE ZONES

In Buettner's third book about Blue Zones, he provides dietary recommendations based on his observations.[**274**] Specifically, he reveals that residents across all Blue Zones consume more beans per day than the rest of us. Buettner promotes beans as a longevity food. He suggests that eating one cup of beans every day will help "... transform any home into a miniature blue zone."

Many health advocates also recommend beans. TR highly recommends beans. It's a staple of the Gatherer diet. But Western society tends to ridicule beans. We make jokes about beans because of what can happen when we eat them.

We're going to need more brave explorers like Buettner to help change the public perception of beans. In this book, we rely on our imagination and, in particular, Imaginary Buettner to make the case for why beans should fuel your blue zone.

Let's imagine how the skills of Imaginary Buettner help him

274 Buettner, D. **The Blue Zones Solution: Eating and Living Like the World's Healthiest People.** National Geographic. 1st edition. April 7, 2015.   *amazon.com/The-Blue-Zones-Solution-Healthiest/dp/1426211929*

sense the unique aura of really old people who eat large quantities of beans. Perhaps it's his sensitive nose. Perhaps it's his sensitive ear. Or perhaps, it's just explorer's instinct.

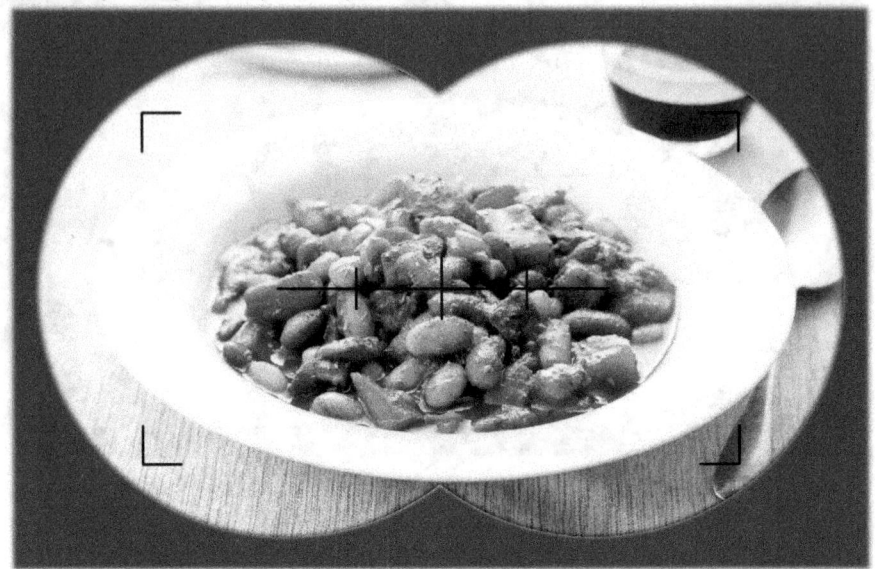

Imaginary Buettner observes one cup of beans is eaten daily in every Blue Zone.

Imaginary Buettner wants us to create our own personal blue zones by eating more beans. He wants to draw a big blue circle around the entire globe.

And we can help him, one cup of beans at a time. Every cup of beans we eat will make our personal blue zone more rich and more potent. It will linger around us and protect us all day long.

If one cup of beans per day can ward off LTDs. Then two cups of beans might ward off actual people with LTDs or frankly anyone with the power of self-locomotion. We'll be safe and protected — in our personal blue zone.

BEANS STIMULATE A DIETARY MOVEMENT

It may seem odd that we don't already have a public advocacy group for fresh beans. We have advocacy groups for other fresh foods such as the National Dairy Council and the National Cattlemen's Beef Association. We regularly hear advertisements promoting fresh milk and fresh beef. But we don't hear advertisements for fresh beans.

We might imagine our forefathers once assembled a National Fresh Bean Council. But when so many bean lovers met in one building, something like a critical mass overwhelmed the ventilation system. Someone had the bright idea of lighting a match to clear the air. That was the last we ever heard of the National Fresh Bean Council.

In its place, we now have a U.S. Dry Bean Council,[**275**] and a USA Dry Pea & Lentil Council.[**276**] These are real organizations, but they have strange names that seem to do a disservice to their products. They advocate for DRY beans, peas, and lentils but not FRESH beans, peas, and lentils. How many consumers find it mouthwatering to think about DRY beans, peas, and lentils?

Perhaps these councils learned from past mistakes and advocate for beans in dry form to safely handle their richness and potency. Perhaps they also divide up the advocacy for dry beans and dry peas to avoid a repeat of the critical mass disaster.

The dry bean and dry pea councils offer the following recipes for us power up our personal blue zones. Don't be alarmed by the recipe names. They're 100% real. They're 100% serious. And they're meant to convey the extraordinary power of the bean.

- *Berry bean blast.*[**277**]
- *Fruity bean logs.*[**278**]
- *Idaho bean fudge.*[**279**]
- *Peanut butter chickpea energy balls.*[**280**]

---

275 U.S. Dry Bean Council website. **Welcome Page.** Accessed 2016. *usdrybeans.com*

276 USA Dry Pea & Lentil Council website. **Welcome Page.** Accessed 2016. *pea-lentil.com*

277 U.S. Dry Bean Council website. **Berry bean blast.** Accessed 2016. *usdrybeans.com/2010/08/berry-bean-blast*

278 U.S. Dry Bean Council website. **Fruity bean logs.** Accessed 2016. *usdrybeans.com/2013/09/fruity-bean-logs*

279 U.S. Dry Bean Council website. **Idaho bean fudge.** Accessed 2016. *usdrybeans.com/2010/08/idaho-bean-fudge*

280 USA Dry Pea & Lentil Council website. **Peanut butter chickpea energy balls.** Accessed 2016. *cookingwithpulses.com/recipes/peanut-butter-chickpea-energy-balls*

We might imagine the dry bean and pea councils setting up a partnership with Imaginary Buettner. The dry bean and pea councils could show us how beans help power up our personal blue zones. Imaginary Buettner could show us how beans help him rocket around the globe.

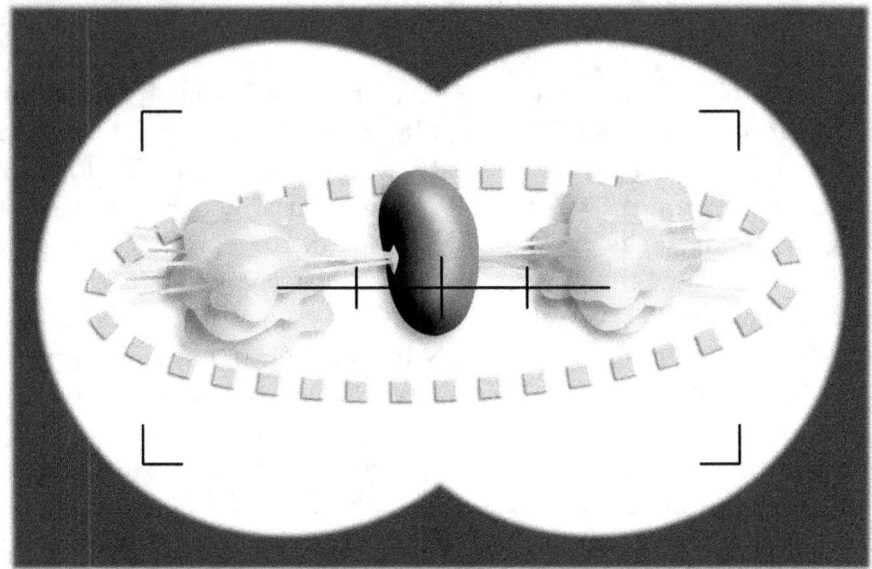

Imaginary Buettner observes a personal Blue Zone.

Consider how the Dairy Council has made "moo-staches" socially acceptable. The cross-marketing relationship could make "personal blue zones" socially acceptable.

We're all familiar with the successful "Got milk?" campaign. The opportunity is ripe for a bean campaign. There are so many catchy slogans we might consider.
- *"Fuel your zone."*
- *"Start a movement."*
- *"Far today, keeps the doctor away."*

BLUE ZONE SPECIAL OPS

The Blue Zone franchise taps into our yearning for discovery and knowledge as we age. We begin contemplating our own mortality. We begin wondering if there might be communities in this world that have figured out health and longevity.

Real Buettner and National Geographic have been very successful with the franchise. It includes best-selling books, films, and industry sponsors. It's a media franchise based on Buettner's expertise as a global explorer.

In honor of the fine work of National Geographic, we create the Imaginary National Geographic for visualization exercises. Imaginary Buettner and Imaginary National Geographic work together like a dream team.

Most of us cannot travel to Blue Zones. Yet we CAN use our imagination to explore them. Better yet, we can follow Imaginary Buettner as he bravely explores communities inhabited by old people who eat lots of beans.

Imaginary Buettner journeys to a purported Blue Zone in an Imaginary National Geographic-chartered plane. He asks the pilot to circle overhead while he straps on his gear. He parachutes to the ground. He establishes an observation post.

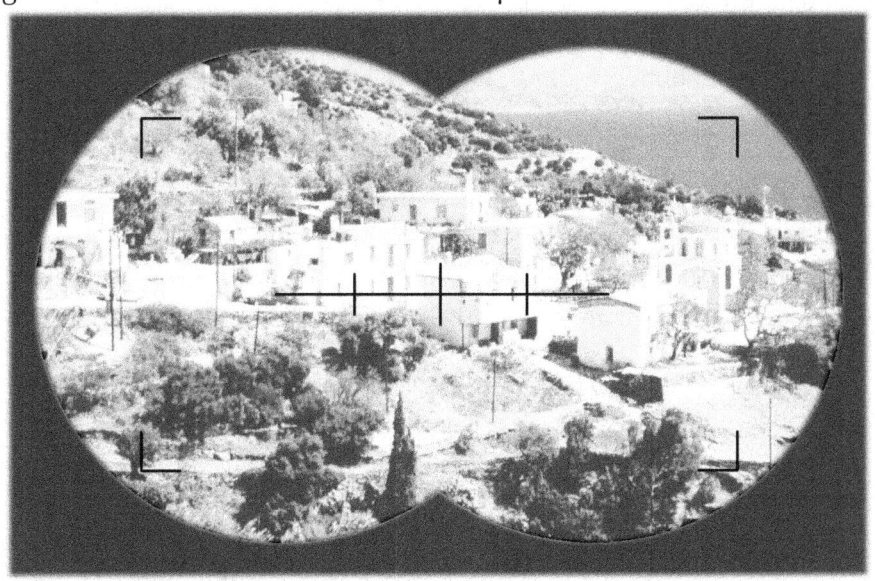

Imaginary Buettner observes an old person community.

He begins monitoring the movements of really old people in their native habitat. He assembles a super-zoom camera and a super-zoom microphone to record his observations.

"Day two of my field study. The one with white crested features is presenting one cup of fresh beans to the one

with spectacled features. This appears to be a daily ritual.
As soon as they enter a noon-time rest phase, I'll move in
closer for measurements."

Imaginary Buettner deciphers their language and establishes communication. This next part requires translation.

"I come from far away. Be not afraid. I want to learn your
ways. I ask to be your student."

"Are you the young fella trying to friend us on social
media?"

Since we're not explorers, we might question why we need to be in such a hustle. These really old people aren't going anywhere. They've been in the same place for a hundred years.

But Imaginary Buettner isn't worried about the Blue Zone residents disappearing. He's worried about the coercive influences of mainstream Western culture, globalization, and Zombie Inc. The sooner he documents their lifestyle, the closer he gets to their native and uncontaminated habits.

BLUE ZONE UNDERCOVER

For fun, we can consider how Imaginary National Geographic has an undercover mission. Imagine the Blue Zone project as a secret geographical survey across planet Earth to find a geologic Fountain of Youth.

A secret geographical survey would explain why these communities are called Blue Zones. The name conveys something special about the location — like there's magic in the water, the soil, or the beans.

The original Blue Zone demographers "claim" the color blue was chosen completely arbitrarily.[281] They "claim" the color blue was chosen simply because they drew blue circles on a map to identify healthy communities.

Might this explanation be a ruse? If they used some other color,

---

281 Poulain M, Pes GM, Grasland C, Carru C, Ferrucci L, Baggio G, Franceschi C, Deiana L. **Identification of a geographic area characterized by extreme longevity in the Sardinia island: the AKEA study.** Exp Gerontol. 2004 Sep;39(9):1423-9. *pubmed.gov/15489066*

such as red, brown, or black, they would have been left with utterly uninspiring names for their zones. Who would ever aspire to live in a Red Zone, a Brown Zone, or a Black Zone? Any media franchise based on Red Zones, Brown Zones, or Black Zones would be a financial flop.

A secret geographical survey is a great backstory to why Imaginary Buettner, an intrepid explorer, is teaming up with Imaginary National Geographic to track old people. He's gathering evidence about their magical soil and their magical beans. Only someone with Imaginary Buettner's skills can get close to a live target and collect biological samples without arousing suspicion.

"Son, why do you keep visiting my bathroom? And why are your pockets bulging?"

A BIG SHOUT OUT

Humor aside, the National Geographic and the Blue Zone team have helped us envision communities where personal health happens naturally. Real Buettner and his Blue Zone team are helping communities here at home.[282] They're setting up private-public partnerships in select cities. They're helping cities build community gardens, pedestrian-friendly walkways, and bike-friendly streets. They're encouraging grocery stores to promote fresh foods.

We should all congratulate Buettner and his Blue Zone team for the great work. They're a real inspiration.

---

282   BlueZones.com. **Services>Built environment.** Accessed 2016. *www. bluezones.com/services/cities*

CHAPTER TEN REVIEW

Blue Zones. These small communities follow a lifestyle that fosters health and longevity. They are scattered across the globe. They tend to lose their unique lifestyles as globalization gains greater influence.

Beans. Dan Buettner, author of the Blue Zones books, has discovered that Blue Zone residents tend to eat a cup of beans per day. He recommends everyone eat one cup of beans every day.

CHAPTER TEN IMAGINE

Imagine we had an organization like the Blue Zone team with even greater ambitions for health activism. It could combine the persistence of Greenpeace with the humor of Comedy Central. Let's imagine it calls itself Code Yellow.

Currently, media coverage of public health bores all of us zombies. Some zombies even get furious about public health, like it's part of a nanny government state. Code Yellow might highlight how Zombie Inc. relies on these anti-government zombies as supporters.

Code Yellow might search for communities with public health interventions that successfully repel the influence of Zombie Inc. Code Yellow might search for communities succumbing to disease caused by the influence of Zombie Inc. We can imagine film footage of Imaginary Buettner traveling for Code Yellow.

> *He encounters a discarded bag of fast food. He carefully opens the bag and smells the contents. He determines what LTD promoting food was eaten. He estimates how much. His jaws clench and his eyes narrow as he casts a penetrating gaze far off toward the horizon.*

Imagine Code Yellow is ambitious enough to take on Zombie Inc. They might document the expanding influence of Zombie Inc. inside our government, our neighborhoods, and in developing countries. They might explain the political and regulatory consequences of the Supreme Court decision of *Citizens United v FEC*. They might explain how Zombie Inc. funds politicians who foment outrage against government regulations. They might explain how Zombie Inc. spreads zombie viruses to angry voters who then vote for anti-government politicians.

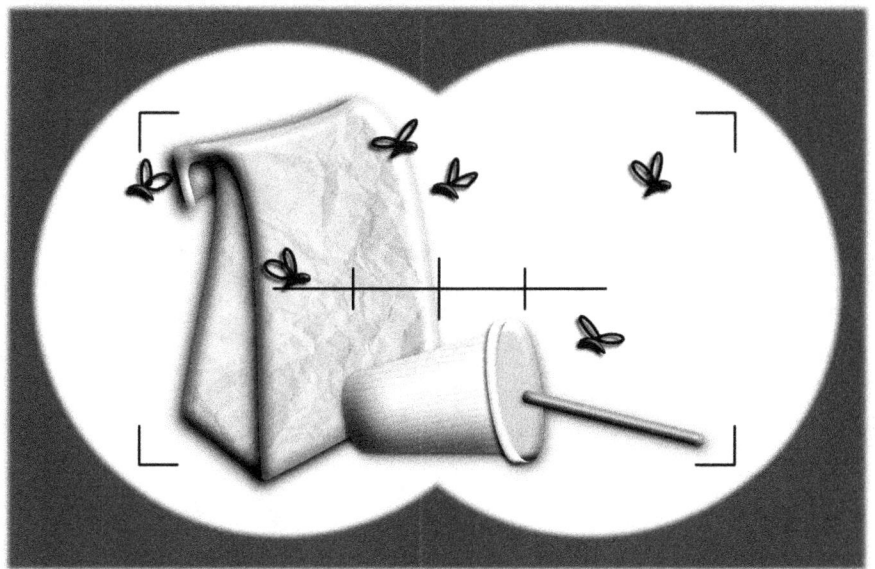

Imaginary Buettner observes a discarded bag of fast food.

We really need an organization to help rally public pressure for more government scrutiny, transparency, and political funding reform. Without an organized opposition, Zombie Inc. will continue to dismantle our government, erode our health, and erode the environment.

ONE MORE THING

As we wrap things up, let's talk about something more personal. Let's talk about YOU and Total Recovery.

Do you remember the day you and TR were first introduced to each other? Are you impressed the relationship has lasted this long? This whole book was like a trial period for the relationship. The two of you made it through, and you're still together.

But the relationship been pretty one-sided.

TR has been doing a lot of talking, and you've been doing a lot of listening. And you've been a great listener. But TR is going to stop talking for a while. Now's your chance to begin doing the talking as you seek greater mindfulness throughout the day.

The next phase of the relationship will depend on you rousing your inner voice. You're going to have to start telling TR about what's going on in your life. Think of it as a mindfulness exercise. Just you and TR, talking about all the emotional stuff. TR will always hang around, but the relationship will get more meaningful the deeper you get. Don't worry, TR can handle it.

Consider how TR has opened your eyes to all the zombies around you. You may be noticing just how much zombie food is for sale at your local grocery stores and restaurants. You may be noticing zombie behaviors in yourself and in the rest of us. You may be noticing what we zombies are doing that age us so fast. You probably see everything differently now, thanks to TR. You probably feel like you're a different person and like the world is a different place now that TR is in your life. You may feel lucky to have met TR.

Consider your own struggles with zombie viruses. Consider keeping a journal of the zombie viruses in your life. Jot down where they come from, what behaviors they cause, and ways to neutralize them. These are the things that TR likes to hear.

Consider whether your health is at risk for any lifestyle trans- mitted diseases. Think through which of your friends and loved ones might need "the talk" about LTDs and about healthy ways to share food and activities with you. Don't worry, TR will be there to back you up in these talks.

Consider how Zombie Inc. is always flirting with you. Take an inventory of all the products and services that bring you short-term happiness, but erode your long-term fitness.

Your relationship with Zombie Inc. is definitely toxic. You'll be much happier to dump Zombie Inc. and focus on TR from now on. Zombie Inc. will keep calling, but just hang up and stop answering. Consider hanging out somewhere else for a while until Zombie Inc. stops looking for you.

Consider all the steps you can take to strengthen the five fit- nesses and recover your biological youth. Don't worry, TR likes to listen to these things too. TR will listen to this stuff forever.

You and TR have a lot of potential together. Think of the rela- tionship as a mindfulness exercise that will last as long as you're willing to put in the effort. And, now it's your turn to help build the relationship.

INDEX

ABOUT THE AUTHOR

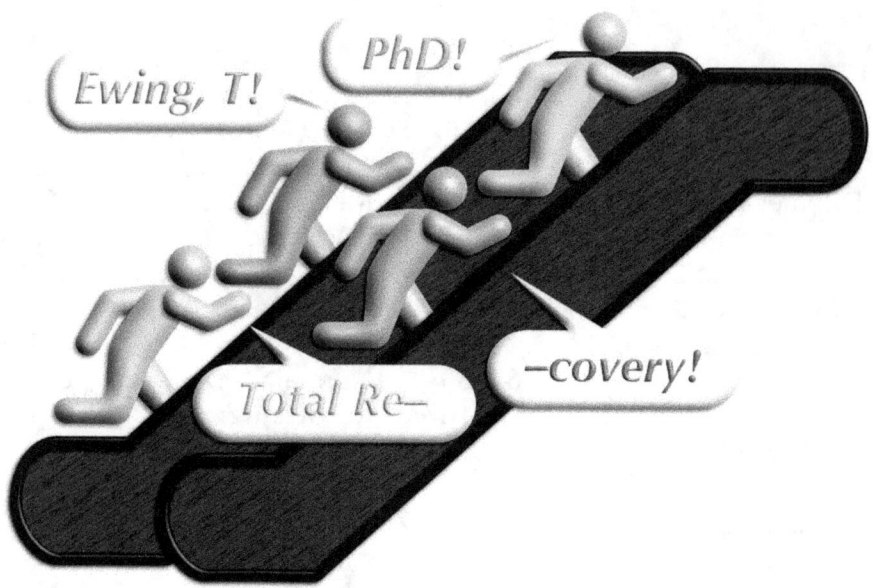

For the past 20 years, Todd Ewing, Ph.D. has dedicated his career to pharmaceutical research while struggling with the belief that a healthy lifestyle is more effective at treating and preventing our deadliest diseases: heart disease, cancer, and Alzheimer's. At the same time, he has struggled with the perception that lifestyles appear to be getting less healthy and people seem to be aging faster. With his new book, Biological Youth, he hopes to spark a revolution in mindfulness, in health and lifestyle awareness, and in the reduction of disease and aging.

Todd Ewing, Ph.D. will follow up Book One: Biological Youth with Book Two: Biological Happiness and many more books in the Total Recovery Series. He hopes each book about Total Recovery will help increase mindfulness, personal health, public health, environmental health, and everything else that is good.

He studied Biology and Chemical Engineering at Stanford University and the University of Washington. He received his Doctorate in Pharmaceutical Sciences from the University of California San Francisco in 1997. He currently resides in the San Francisco Bay Area.